Advanced aspects of imaging in oral implantology

Arthur Rodriguez Gonzalez Cortes

ISBN: 1515311503
ISBN-13: 978-1515311508

Dedication

This book is dedicated to my wife, Juliana, who has supported my every endeavor; to my son, Eric, of whom I'm so proud and thankful; to my brother Thomaz, who is one of my main inspirations; and to my parents Djalma and Carmen, who have supported all my ideas.

About the Editor and Contributors

Editor

Arthur Rodriguez Gonzalez Cortes, DDS, PhD.
Postdoctoral Research Fellow, Martinos Center for Biomedical Imaging, Department of Radiology, Massachusetts General Hospital, Charlestown, MA, USA; Postdoctoral Research Fellow, Department of Radiology, Harvard Medical School, Boston, MA, USA.

Contributors

Claudio Costa, DDS, PhD.
Associate Professor, Oral Radiology Division, School of Dentistry, University of Sao Paulo, Sao Paulo, Brazil.

Gilberto Araujo Noro Filho, DDS, MS.
PhD student, Oral Radiology Division, School of Dentistry, University of Sao Paulo, Sao Paulo, Brazil; Adjunt Professor, School of Dentistry, Paulista University, Sao Paulo, Brazil.

Emiko Saito Arita, DDS, PhD.
Associate Professor, Oral Radiology Division, School of Dentistry, University of Sao Paulo, Sao Paulo, Brazil.

Jerome L. Ackerman, PhD.
Director, Biomaterials Laboratory, Martinos Center for Biomedical Imaging, Massachusetts General Hospital, Charlestown, MA, USA; Associate Professor of Radiology, Harvard Medical School.

Jorge de Sá Barbosa, DDS, PhD.
Assistant Professor, School of Dentistry, Metropolitan University of Santos, Santos, SP, Brazil.

José Marcio Barbosa Leite do Amaral, DDS, MS.
Professor, School of Dentistry, Metropolitan University of Santos, Santos, SP, Brazil.

Lucas Rodrigues Pinheiro, DDS, PhD.
Private practice, Belém, PA, Brazil.

Jesus Torres García-Denche, DDS, PhD.
Assistant Professor, Faculty of Dentistry, Complutense University, Madrid, Spain.

Faleh Tamimi, BDS, PhD.
Assistant Professor, Faculty of Dentistry, McGill University, Montreal, Canada.

Djalma Nogueira Cortes, DDS.
Private practice, Sao Paulo, SP, Brazil.

CONTENTS

Acknowledgments 6

1 *Planning an implant therapy:* 7
Review of basic concepts
Claudio Costa, Gilberto Araujo Noro Filho &
Arthur Rodriguez Gonzalez Cortes

2 *Assessment of the alveolar bone tissue* 17
Arthur Rodriguez Gonzalez Cortes, Emiko
Saito Arita & Jerome L. Ackerman

3 **Image-guided implant surgery** 30
Jorge de Sá Barbosa, José Marcio Barbosa
Leite do Amaral & Arthur Rodriguez Gonzalez Cortes

4 **Dental implant follow-up** 37
Lucas Rodrigues Pinheiro &
Arthur Rodriguez Gonzalez Cortes

5 **Lateral ridge augmentation:** 47
Particulate bone grafts
Arthur Rodriguez Gonzalez Cortes

6 **Block Bone grafts** 52
Jesus Torres García-Denche, Faleh Tamimi &
Arthur Rodriguez Gonzalez Cortes

7 **Sinus floor augmentation** 63
Arthur Rodriguez Gonzalez Cortes &
Djalma Nogueira Cortes

ACKNOWLEDGEMENTS

The Editor would like to thank The National Council for Research and Development of Brazil (CNPq) for supporting his postdoctoral fellowship at Harvard Medical School, Boston, MA, USA. The editor would also like to thank the other contributors for their willing support. Finally, the editor would like to thank the following institutions for their support: University of Sao Paulo, Sao Paulo, Brazil; Metropolitan University of Santos, Santos, SP, Brazil; McGill University, Montreal, Canada; Harvard Medical School, Boston, MA, USA; and Martinos Center of Biomedical Imaging, Massachusetts General Hospital, Charlestown, MA, USA.

CHAPTER 1

PLANNING AN IMPLANT THERAPY: REVIEW OF BASIC CONCEPTS

Claudio Costa
Giberto Araujo Noro Filho
Arthur Rodriguez Gonzalez Cortes

Diagnostic imaging is the primary stage in the development of integrated treatment plans for rehabilitation with dental implants. Radiographic images can be used to identify and locate vital anatomical structures, as well as to get detailed information on the remaining alveolar bone tissue, including measurements of length and thickness. It is also possible to perform bone qualitative analysis before implant installation.

Each radiographic technique has a different application in surgical and/or prosthetic planning. Multiple factors will influence the selection of the most appropriate radiographic technique, including procedure type, cost, availability, radiation exposure, and patient's anatomical variations.[1]

In first place, the optimal implant position should be evaluated considering three important spatial planes: mesiodistal, buccolingual and apicocoronal. Furthermore, regardless of which techniques are being used, the radiographic examination should always follow a detailed clinical examination, in order to develop an adequate therapeutic management.

Each radiographic technique provides a different view of the remaining alveolar bone tissue, with varying degrees of magnification and/or distortion. Therefore, the decision on the type of radiographic image to be used for planning an implant therapy must take into account various factors such as number of dental implant sites, degree of bone resorption, presence of bone grafts and image accuracy. Radiation doses to the patients should be in accordance with the principles of the "as low as reasonably achievable" (ALARA) guidelines.[2]

Due to constant technological development of diagnostic image-obtaining methods and computer programs, ongoing improvement and professional updates are of fundamental importance to health professionals, especially those working with dental implants, to achieve the elaboration of an integrated treatment plan, appropriate for each individual case.

Radiographic Techniques

Periapical radiography

The periapical techniques provide two-dimensional (2D) images, allowing for subjective assessment of remaining alveolar bone.[3] The most used method in oral implantology is the paralleling technique. It minimizes distortions, despite not eliminating them, since distortion is inherent to the process of formation of this type of radiographic image. This technique is useful to perform an assessment of the periodontal status of nearby teeth, preliminary determination of vertical height of small edentulous regions and implant follow-up (Figure 1-1).[1]

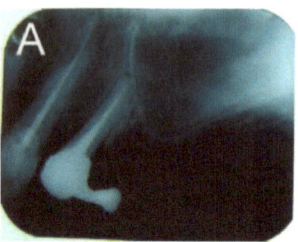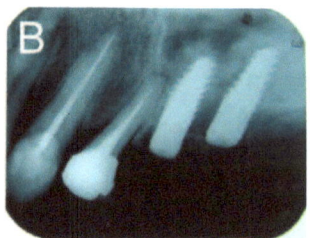

Figure 1-1. *Pre- (A) and postoperative (B) periapical radiographs.*

Periapical radiographs are also well-suited for the intrasurgical evaluation of dental implant placement procedures (Figure 1-2). Radiographs can be taken after flap opening, implant site drilling and stationing of the parallel pin, in order to ensure the satisfactory execution of the surgical plan.[4]

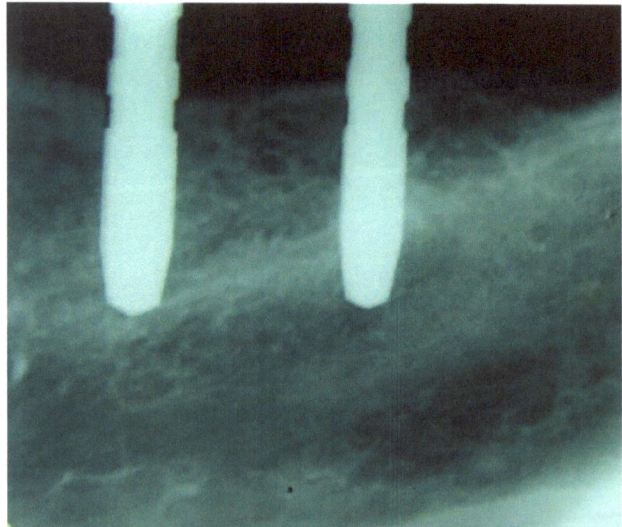

Figure 1-2. *Radiographic view of two parallel pins, ensuring satisfactory implant placement conditions.*

Occlusal radiography

Occlusal radiography is a 2D examination, in which the x-ray beam is oblique (usually 45 to 65 degrees) to the film for obtaining maxillary images and perpendicular to the film for obtaining mandibular images. In both cases, the film is placed parallel to the occlusal plane. Occlusal radiographic images are useful for screening pathologies throughout the alveolar ridge. Anatomical structures such as the maxillary sinus, nasal cavity, and nasopalatine canal can be assessed with this technique, but with no precise spatial relationship. In addition, it does not allow for the visualization of the maxillary cortical bone. Although the mandibular cortical bone is clearly visible, it is not possible to perform accurate measurements of the mandibular buccolingual width in a single axial plane, because of the concomitant presence of the inferior mandibular cortex in the image.[1]

Lateral cephalometric projection

Lateral cephalometric projections, also named lateral cephalometric radiographs, are obtained with the patient's midsagittal plane oriented parallel to the film. The images are magnified and allow for the observation of the buccolingual extension of anterior regions of both maxilla and mandible, insofar this technique presents only small distortions. It can also be used as a guide to evaluate vertical dimension. In addition, lateral cephalometric radiographs can also be taken with a 45-degree angle to the midsagittal plane (lateral-oblique cephalometric radiographs). The aforementioned technique was widely used in the decade of 80's to measure bone height and thickness at premolar and molar sites.[5] The main disadvantages of lateral cephalometric radiographs are that the images do not allow for assessments of bone quality, and only one cross-sectional image of the alveolar bone is offered to assess edentulous sites where the central beam of x-rays is tangent to the ridge (Figure 1-3).

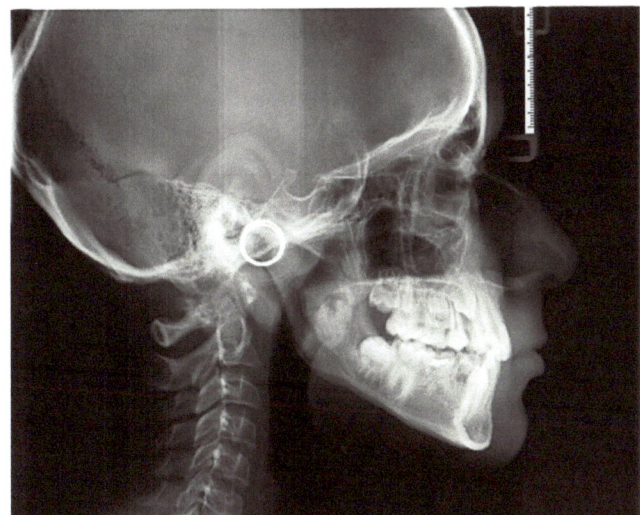

Figure 1-3. *Lateral cephalometric projection.*

Panoramic radiography

In the past, 2D panoramic radiographs were the most commonly used radiographic examination in the preoperative diagnosis and planning of dental implants. The images depict the entire maxillary and mandibular bodies in a curved plane, and are easy to interpret. Panoramic radiographs are indicated to assess opposing landmarks and vertical height of the ridge (Figure 1-4). On the other hand, the images have varying degrees of magnification. The horizontal magnification follows a logarithmic equation, being higher at the posterior regions (It may reach around 60% in the condyle area). However, the vertical magnification is lower, with values oscillating around an average over the entire film, since it follows a linear equation. As a result, panoramic radiographs cannot be used for accurate measurements of the remaining bone thickness or direct measurements of alveolar bone density. In addition, vertical measurements made in panoramic radiographs of atrophic maxillae may understate the remaining alveolar bone height, in contrast with the high accuracy of computed tomographic scans.[6]

Linear tomography

Linear tomography (also commonly referred to as conventional tomography) is a widely accessible radiographic technique used for the cross-sectional imaging of edentulous jaws (Figure 1-5), and is relatively inexpensive compared with computed tomography. In addition, linear tomography offers less radiation doses to the patient than a computed tomographic scan when used to image a single site.[7]

Linear tomography is based on the synchronized movement between x-ray source and image receptor. The images have a balanced degree of magnification and no distortions, provided that the method fulfills certain technical criteria. As a result, it is possible to measure the alveolar ridge height and thickness accurately, and to perform analyses of the bone density using subjective classifications.[8] With the development of tomographic systems, there has been an improvement in the image quality and consequently in the depiction of several important anatomical details.

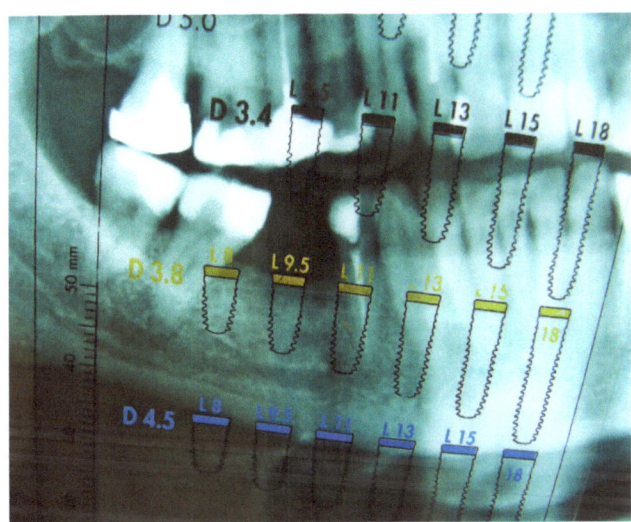

Figure 1-4. *A transparent ruler (DENTSPLY-Friadent, Mannheim, Germany) was used for planning an implant placement on a panoramic radiographic image.*

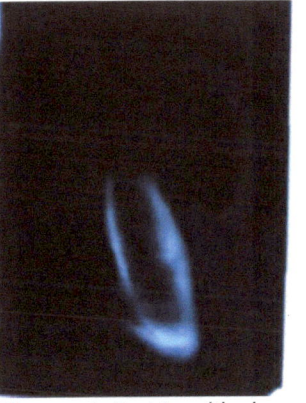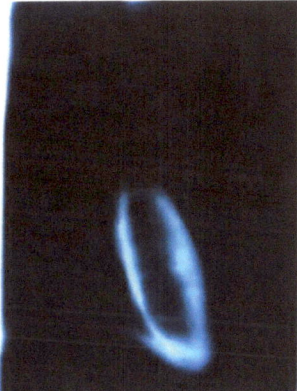

Figure 1-5. *Mandibular cross-sectional images from linear tomography.*

Computed tomography

Computed tomography (CT) was invented and introduced by Sir Godfrey Hounsfield in 1972. It is a digital radiographic examination that does not present significant image magnification or distortion, allowing the professional to perform accurate measurements of the alveolar ridge height and thickness. With this method, it is also possible to carry out quantitative analyses of the bone density by using the Hounsfield scale. The indication of this examination must meet the selection criteria outlined by the American Academy of Oral and Maxillofacial Radiology, as well as the principles of ALARA[2] in order to control the radiation dose levels received by the patient. Computed tomographic images are digitally reconstructed from the raw data acquired by using algorithms. The smallest component of the digital image is the pixel (picture elements).

Each pixel is assigned a CT number (related to the x-ray attenuation of the tissue), commonly referred as Hounsfield units. Pixels are grouped and reformatted into three-dimensional (3D) models composed by volume elements, named voxels. The voxel size will depend on the pixel size and on the slice thickness. In general, smaller voxels lead to a better image quality. CT Images are usually provided in the DICOM (Digital Imaging Communication in Medicine) format.

There are two main types of computed tomography: Medical CT (or spiral CT) and cone beam CT (CBCT).

Medical CT uses a thin and collimated "fan beam" of x-rays that rotates around the patient. Considering a single detector helical CT device, only one slice is acquired per revolution. Therefore, the scanning time is long and the radiation doses received by the patient are high. However, high-contrast images can be produced and used for bone density quantitative analyses (Figure 1-6).

Cone beam CT was developed and adapted for the dental purposes. It uses a flat-panel detector to acquire all x-ray projections required to reconstruct the volume in only one rotation. Therefore, the scanning time is shorter and the effective radiation doses received by the patient are lower compared to the medical CT.

CBCT Images can be reconstructed in any plane with an acceptable contrast resolution (Figure 7). X-ray scatter correction using algorithms can be useful in order to improve CBCT image quality. Compared with other CT methods, CBCT offers advantages such as reduced effective radiation doses, easier imaging, shorter acquisition scan times, and lower costs.[9]

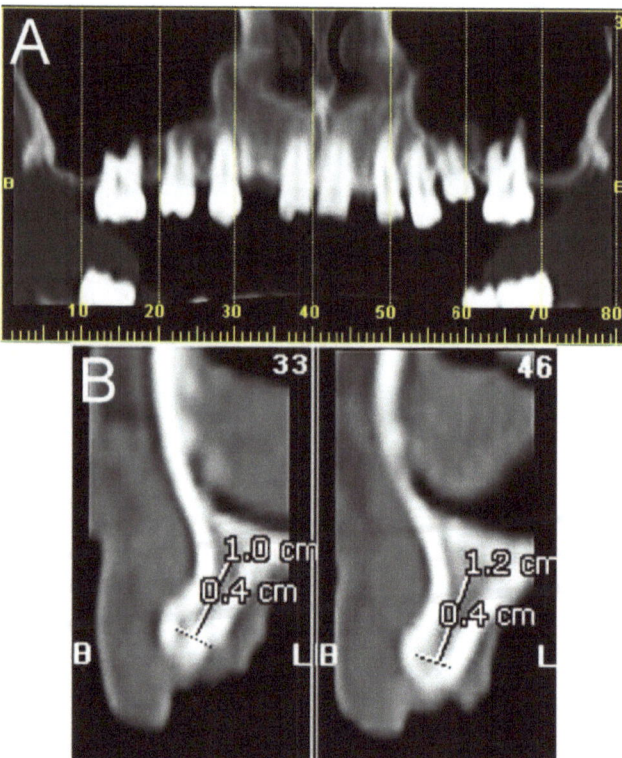

Figure 1-6. *Medical CT images. A) Coronal panoramic cut. B) Cross-sectional images of the edentulous sites.*

A summary of the differences between medical CT and CBCT can be found in the table 1.

Table 1-1. Differences between CT and CBCT

	CT	CBCT
Scanning time	Longer	Shorter
Radiation doses	Higher	Lower
Contrast	Higher	Lower
Main indication	Hard and soft tissues	Hard tissues
Positioning	Sensitive	Not an issue
Design	Hospital	In-office
Cost	Higher	Lower
Availability	Lower	Higher

Working with CBCT images

Printed X Digital CBCT images for implant surgical planning

With the advent of CBCT on implant dentistry, printed CBCT images with schematic drawings (usually made by oral and maxillofacial radiologists) have been used to orientate oral surgeons (Figure 1-7). Optimal dental implant positions can be chosen according to both the condition of the underlying bone assessed in cross-sectional images and the prosthetic rehabilitation plan. However, this method involves waste of chemicals and printed materials. In addition, because it is not possible to navigate through and control the different orthogonal planes at the same time, no true three-dimensional analysis can be done. In other words, instead of the entire volume, it is a group of 2D slices that are individually analyzed.

On the other hand, CT computer softwares allow for an interactive analysis of all orthogonal planes, which may improve dental implant planning. By using 3D multiplanar reconstructions that are generated from CBCT data, the professional can navigate through three orthogonal planes (axial, sagittal, coronal) and a curved plane (coronal panoramic) at the same time. In the most used software interfaces, each window shows a different rotatable plane and has two different guides (axis) respective to the other two planes. This allows the professional to perform a 3D assessment of the dental implant site. Moreover, implants can be virtually placed in the bone and their 3D positions can be refined and optimized in the multiplanar reconstruction. Then, 3D reconstructed models can be created and the prosthetic result can be instantly predicted. A surgical guide that allows for precise drilling of the virtually planned implant position can also be generated (see chapter 3).

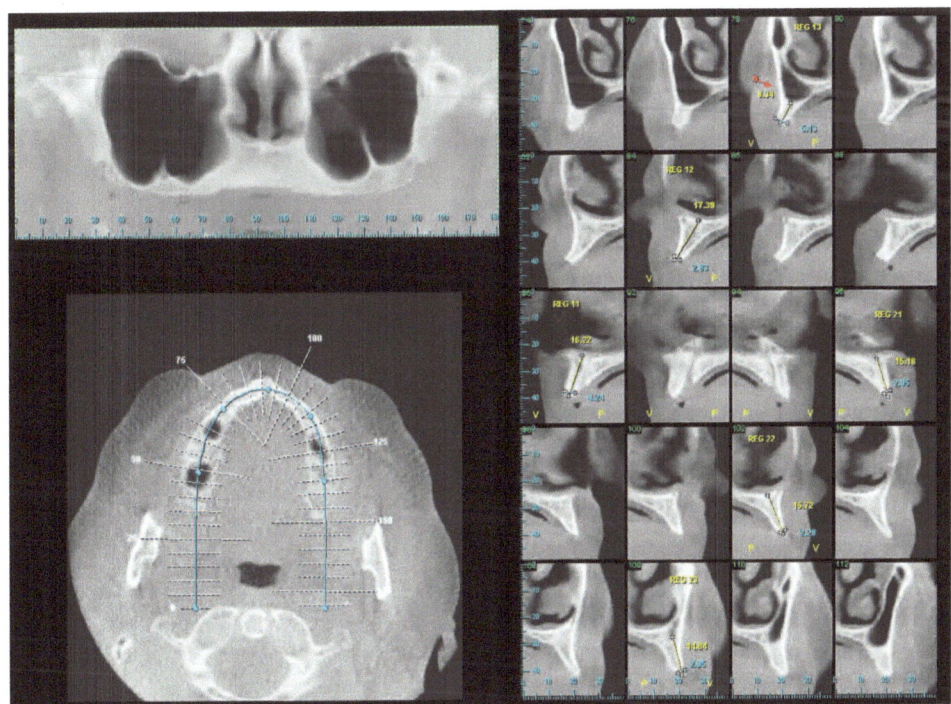

Figure1-7. *Common presentation of CBCT scans printed on films. Cross-sectional images are numbered according to the ruler available on the coronal panoramic image.*

Implant planning softwares

Computer softwares dedicated to oral implantology, such as DentaScan (General Electric Medical Systems, Milwaukee, WI, USA) or ImplantViewer (AnneSolutions, Sao Paulo, Brazil), are designed to evaluate implant sites from axial, cross-sectional (commonly referred as parasagittal in the literature) and coronal panoramic cuts. Three-dimensional images of reconstructed models are also offered in a separate window. This type of software has a user-friendly interface and usually presents tools for linear measurement, gray-scale analysis and virtual implant positioning. Dental implants can be virtually placed, positioned and viewed in all different planes. Some softwares also have tools to predict the prosthetic result, and even to export the results to generate a stereolithographic surgical template (see chapter 3).

Despite the above-mentioned advantages, softwares dedicated to oral implantology are frequently limited in terms of 3D features and tools. Some of these softwares cannot read DICOM files. Instead, the software manufacturer must previously convert the DICOM files to a specific file extension. In addition, sagittal and coronal windows are frequently not available in implant planning softwares. Instead, cross-sectional images are only available along the curved plane of the coronal panoramic window.

In the majority of the cases, these cross-sectional images cannot be freely tilted or rotated. As a result, tilted objects in the image may be depicted in different cross-sectional slices (Figure 1-8).

Radiology softwares

In contrast with implant planning softwares, DICOM viewers dedicated to medical imaging diagnosis and radiology research offer various 3D post-processing protocols and tools. One of the available examples is the OsiriX software (Pixmeo, Geneva, Switzerland). This is an open-source imaging software that can also be used for the diagnosis of dental related treatments,[10,11] including dental implant planning (it requires the installation of a specific plug-in). The three orthogonal planes (axial, sagittal and coronal) can be freely rotated in different windows to provide cross-sectional images of any plane (Figure 1-9). Coronal panoramic cuts can also be generated. In addition, linear, angular and volume measurements (e.g. tissue 3D segmentation) can be performed. Maximum Intensity Projection (MIP) protocols can also be used for diagnosis. Finally, 3D reconstruction models can be created and enhanced with threshold color edition, which allows for the visualization of more anatomical structures in a 3D model with high image quality (Figure 1-10).

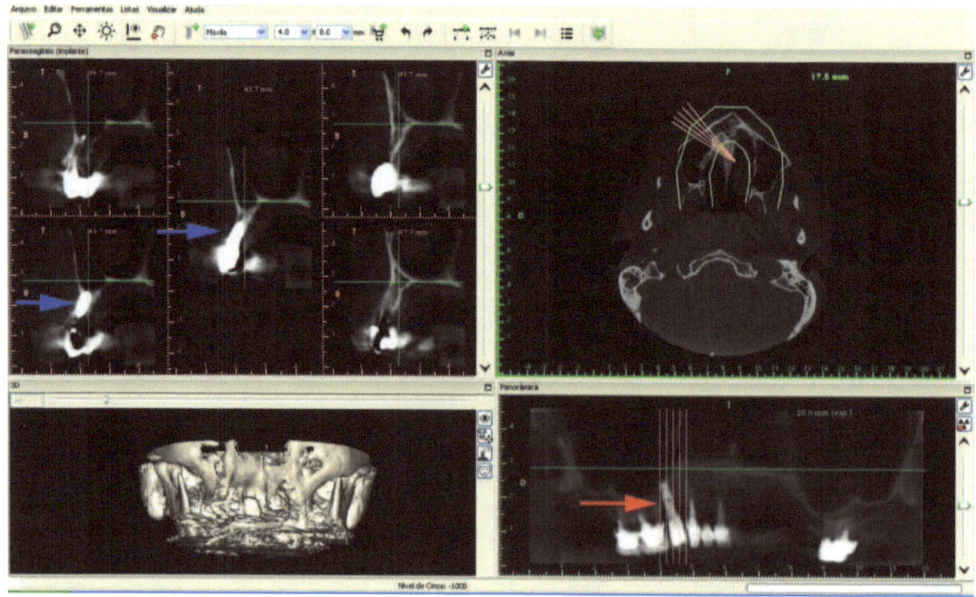

Figure 1-8. *Screenshot of the ImplantViewer software. A distally tilted implant (red arrow) was depicted in different cross-sectional slices (blue arrows).*

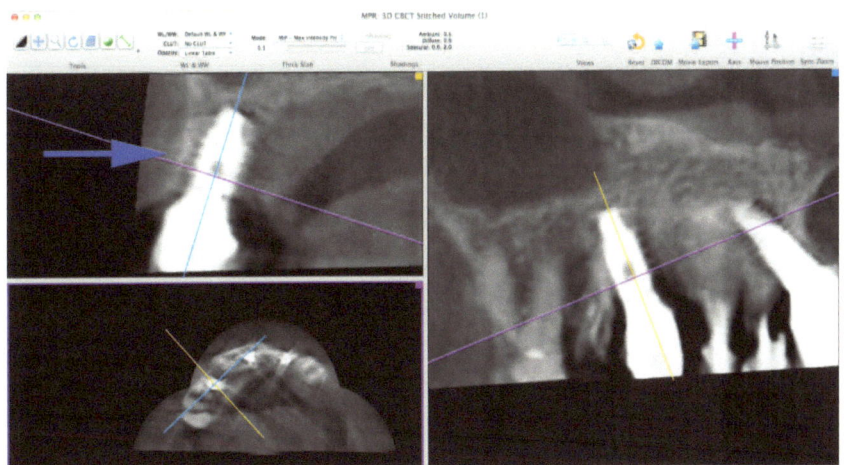

Figure 1-9. *Screenshot of the OsiriX software. A distally tilted implant could be entirely depicted in only one cross-sectional slice (blue arrow).*

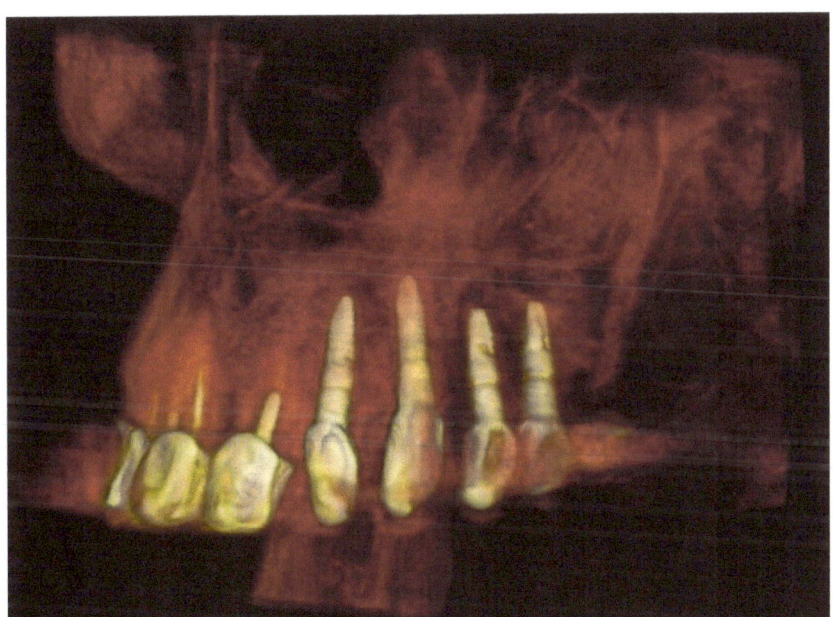

Figure 1-10. *3D-CBCT reconstructed image of maxilla after threshold color edition. High contrasts select either metallic bodies or bone density, while low contrasts select soft tissue contours and spaces.*

How does "threshold color edition" work?

The rendering algorithm of the software assigns a given color and opacity to the lowest level of intensity displayed. This allows setting the rendering of different tissue densities (skin, muscle or bones). The program assigns a color and opacity to each of the contrast and intensity levels included in the tomography.

Therefore, the professional can edit some of the characteristics of 3D reconstruction models. Contrast and intensity are two factors responsible for selecting the threshold density value used for rendering the opaque tissue level.

Threshold levels can also be used to accurately digitize radiographic guides, so that 3D models can be created using optimal thresholds.[12] Further studies would also be recommended to assess other clinical applications of this method.

CT Applications for mobile devices

Tablets and smartphones are important innovations in computing technology that have already been incorporated into professional healthcare.[13] Some important characteristics of these devices as potential tools in diagnostic medicine include small size, web access, touch screen display, satisfactory processor performance and screen resolution.

Several studies have reported the suitability of using some mobile devices in a number of medical fields, for such activities as reviewing brain scans,[14] conducting emergency identification of pulmonary embolism,[15] following up on lung surgery,[16] making spinal cord assessments,[17] and diagnosing acute appendicitis.[18] In dentistry, they have already been used to evaluate interproximal caries.[19] Picture Archiving and Communication Systems (PACS) possess the ability to store CT images in DICOM format with high-speed network connectivity, allowing for the timely dissemination of full-resolution medical images with a computer, a mobile device and network connectivity. The location of the aforementioned devices may be within the same facility in which the images are acquired, in remote hospitals or even private dental offices.[13-17]

A recent study[20] used CBCT images provided from files of DICOM format, and manipulated in order to obtain and navigate through 3D multiplanar reconstructions. The OsiriX application for mobile devices was installed in an iPad (Apple, Cuppertino, CA) and in an iPhone, and then linked to the DICOM database server, by connecting both mobile device and workstation to the same wireless network. This enables the mobile devices to receive DICOM images from the workstation database and to open and navigate through images from 3D multiplanar reconstructions.

In the same study,[20] images rendered in the iPad were manipulated during implant placement procedures by a duly trained professional in OsiriX software, in order to follow up and confirm the virtual graft and implant planning at the chairside. The iPad was completely involved in a sterile package so that the surgeon could manipulate it using sterile gloves (Figure 1-11). To send the images to the ipad, the CBCT cross-sectional slice of the implant site was identified in the workstation computer, marked as a region of interest (ROI), and exported to the OsiriX iPad application.

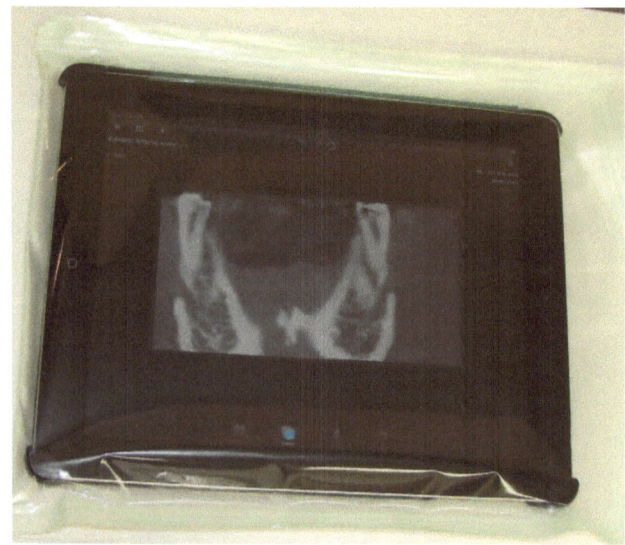

Figure 1-11. *Ipad used during implant surgery.*

OsiriX application for mobile devices provides the function of gray scale analyses using pixel values, as well as both area and linear measurements. Image zooming and rotating can be done by pinching the screen, whereas the level of contrast and brightness can be adjusted by swiping the finger across the display. Since the CBCT cross-sectional slice that corresponds to the implant site is marked as a region of interest (ROI), the surgeon is able to double check and re-measure alveolar bone dimensions during the surgery by performing multi-touch gestures.[20] Despite the above mentioned advantages, only two different CT planes (among parasagittal, sagittal, coronal, axial, or coronal panoramic options) can be examined simultaneously.

In addition, this platform allows the clinician to share images with other professionals by using internet connection, in order to discuss and improve treatment planning based on CT images.[21] Remote access from portable devices to the database server of the image is an important feature that could be useful in dental clinics to provide multiple accesses to a single database server. This kind of interaction among multiple healthcare professionals improves networking. In addition, it is noteworthy that these communication features can be explored in teaching activities related to oral radiology. This technology would allow for faster diagnosis with radiographic examinations, and would reduce the cost of printing CT scans and acquiring hardware equipment.

References

1. Nagarajan A, Perumalsamy R, Thyagarajan R, Namasivayam A. Diagnostic Imaging for Dental Implant Therapy. J Clin Imaging Sci 2014;4:4.
2. Dykstra BA. ALARA and radiation in the dental office: current state of affair. Dent Today 2011;30: 14, 16, 18.
3. Tydall DA, Brooks SL. Selection criteria for dental implant site imaging: a position paper of the American Academy of Oral and Maxillofacial Radiology. Oral Surg Oral Med Oral Pathol Oral Radiol Endod, 2000; 89(5):630-7.
4. Cortes AR. The Importance of Taking Periapical Radiographs during Implant Placement. Implant News & Views, 2012; 14: 1-4.
5. Gröndahl K, Ekestubbe A, Gröndahl HG. Radiography in oral endosseous prosthetics. Gotemborg:Nobel Biocare AB, 1996
6. Fortin T, Camby E, Alik M, Michel Isidori M, Bouchet H. Panoramic images versus three-dimensional planning software for oral implant planning in atrophied posterior maxillary: a clinical radiological study. Clin Implant Dent Relat Res. 2013;15(2):198-204.
7. Dula K, Mini R, van der Stelt PF, Buser D. The radiographic assessment of implant patients: decision-making criteria. Int J Oral Maxillofac Implants. 2001;16:80-9.
8. Misch CE. Contemporary implant dentistry 2nd edn. St Louis, MO: Mosby, 1999.
9. Hirsch E, Wolf U, Heinicke F, Silva MA. Dosimetry of the cone beam computed tomography Veraviewepocs 3D compared with the 3D Accuitomo in different field of views. Dentomaxillofac Radiol. 2008;37:268-73.
10. Cortes AR, Pinheiro LR, Umetsubo OS, Arita ES, Cavalcanti MG. Assessment of implant-related treatment with edited three-dimensional reconstructed images from cone-beam computerized tomography: a technical note. J Oral Implantol. 2014;40:729-32.
11. Costa FF, Gaia BF, Umetsubo OS, Paraiso Cavalcanti MG. Detection of horizontal root fracture with small-volume cone-beam computed tomography in the presence and absence of intracanal metallic post. J Endod 2011:37:1456-9.
12. Wouters V, Mollemans W, Schutyser F. Calibrated segmentation of CBCT and CT images for digitization of dental prostheses. Int J Comput Assist Radiol Surg 2011:6:609-16.
13.Garritty C, El Emam K. Who's using PDAs? estimates of PDA use by health care providers: a systematic review of surveys. J Med Internet Res 2006; 8:e7.
14. Mc Laughlin P, Neill SO, Fanning N, Mc Garrigle AM, Connor OJ, Wyse G, Maher MM. Emergency CT brain: preliminary interpretation with a tablet device: image quality and diagnostic performance of the Apple iPad. Emerg Radiol 2012; 19:127-33.

15. Johnson PT, Zimmerman SL, Heath D, Eng J, Horton KM, Scott WW, Fishman EK. The iPad as a mobile device for CT display and interpretation: diagnostic accuracy for identification of pulmonary embolism. Emerg Radiol 2012; 19:323-7.

16. Volonté F, Robert JH, Ratib O, Triponez F. A lung segmentectomy performed with 3D reconstruction images available on the operating table with an iPad. Interact Cardiovasc Thorac Surg 2011; 12:1066-8.

17. McNulty JP(1), Ryan JT, Evanoff MG, Rainford LA. Flexible image evaluation: iPad versus secondary-class monitors for review of MR spinal emergency cases, a comparative study. Acad Radiol 2012; 19:1023-8.

18. Choudhri AF, Carr TM 3rd, Ho CP, Stone JR, Gay SB, Lambert DL. Handheld device review of abdominal CT for the evaluation of acute appendicitis. J Digit Imaging 2012; 25:492-6.

19. Shintaku WH, Scarbecz M, Venturin JS. Evaluation of interproximal caries using the iPad 2 and a liquid crystal display monitor. .Oral Surg Oral Med Oral Pathol Oral Radiol. 2012;113(5):e40-4

20. Aoki EM; Cortes AR; Arita ES. The use of a CT application for mobile devices in the diagnosis of oral and maxillofacial surgeries: a technical report. J Craniofac Surg, 2015;26(1):e18-e21.

21. Székely A, Talanow R, Bágyi P. Smartphones, tablets and mobile applications for radiology. Eur J Radiol 2013; 82:829-36.

CHAPTER 2

ASSESSMENT OF THE ALVEOLAR BONE TISSUE

Arthur Rodriguez Gonzalez Cortes
Emiko Saito Arita
Jerome L. Ackerman

Despite the continuous development of multiple surgical techniques in oral implantology, severe bone resorption may represent a challenge for the professional to rehabilitate the edentulous jaws. In this context, alveolar ridge bone atrophy has been regarded as an important limiting factor for the success of an implant surgery.[1]

Conditions such as loss of buccal alveolar plate, decreased ridge width and pneumatization of the maxillary sinus are primarily found in partially or fully edentulous jaws. These factors may be presented as contraindications to the placement of implants with conventional techniques.[2] In such cases, placement of bone grafts may be required to achieve treatment success.[3]

Relationship between alveolar bone tissue and implant therapy outcomes

A successful osseointegration of the dental implant depends mainly on the amount and density of bone available in the alveolar ridge, and primary stability. The latter is defined as the lack of mobility of the implant after it is installed in the bone tissue of the implantation site.[4] Primary stability, in turn, depends on the implant insertion torque.[5]

Thus, an adequate insertion torque is crucial to prevent micromotion of the implant, which would lead to failure of osseointegration process, and consequently to loss of the implant.[6]

Furthermore, high implant insertion torque values are recommended for the application of immediate loading, whereby the prosthetic rehabilitation of the patient can be completed immediately after surgical placement of the dental implant, leading to shorter treatment times.[7]

Implant insertion torque is influenced by factors such as surgical technique, implant dimensions and characteristics of the alveolar bone.[5,8] However, only a few methods of quantitative analysis of alveolar bone were correlated or associated with the implant peak insertion torque in the literature. Quantitative analyses on CT images started to be developed and used for the diagnosis of implant surgeries. Such methods showed satisfactory accuracy and precision to measure bone density of the residual ridge.[9] However, these methods do not provide sufficient resolution to resolve the trabecular bone structure. Histological and morphometric analyses, in turn, have the important disadvantage that they cannot be applied in vivo. Moreover, the results of quantitative analyzes in CT images are strongly affected by beam-hardening artifacts caused by presence of metal components in the field of view. This could prevent the radiographic diagnosis of stable dental implants.[10,11]

With the advent of CBCT in oral implantology, there were an increasing number of researches that could help to understand the relationship that exists between features of the alveolar bone and implant stability. Furthermore, different radiographic bone classifications and indices were created and studied.

Panoramic radiomorphometric indices

Since panoramic radiography is a common initial examination at the patient's first attendance, a number of quantitative and qualitative panoramic radiographic measurements were developed and correlated to systemic bone mineral density. These two-dimensional measurements were introduced as radiomorphometric indices, and presented strong correlations with the gold standard values of bone mineral density obtained with bone densitometry.

Among the most evaluated indices are the mandibular cortical width (MCW), corresponding to the cortical thickness of the lower jaw in a line below the mental foramen, perpendicular to a tangent to the lower border of the mandible;[12] and the mandibular cortical index (MCI), which evaluates the radiographic appearance of the inferior mandibular cortex below the mental foramen in a qualitative scale (Figures 2-1 and 2-2).[13,14] It has been suggested that the panoramic radiography should be used routinely as a diagnostic tool for osteoporosis in elderly patients.

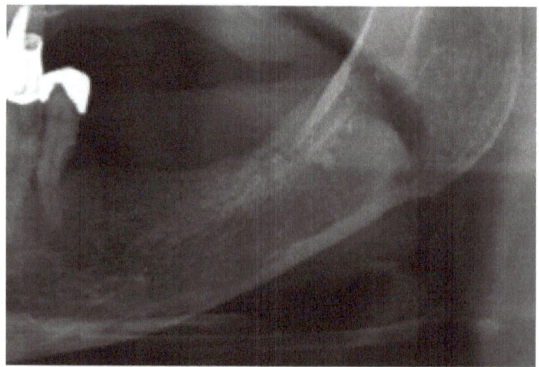

Figure 2-2. *Severely eroded appearance of the inferior mandibular cortex (MCI=C3).*

Another study performed on patients diagnosed with osteoporosis compared results of both MCI and MCW with the expression of biochemical markers of bone turnover.[17] Risk association analysis by odds ratio concluded that there was a strong association between the MCI and alkaline phosphatase levels. However, there was no significant association between the MCW and the same biochemical markers.

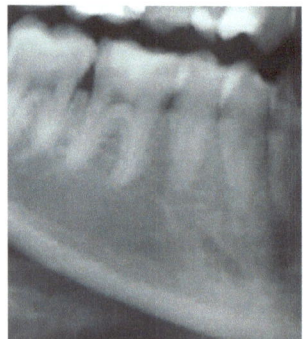

Figure 2-1. *Normal appearance of the inferior mandibular cortex (MCI=C1).*

The above-mentioned indices, as well as systemic bone mineral density assessed with dual x-ray absorptiometry (DXA) were also correlated with alveolar bone resorption rates.[15,16] Imirzalioglu and collaborators[15] evaluated MCI and MCW (Figure 2-3) in 1863 panoramic radiographs of patients, comparing the results obtained with alveolar bone loss levels. There was also a significant correlation between both analyzed indices and patients' age. The authors suggested that both indices could be useful in the diagnosis of alveolar bone loss.

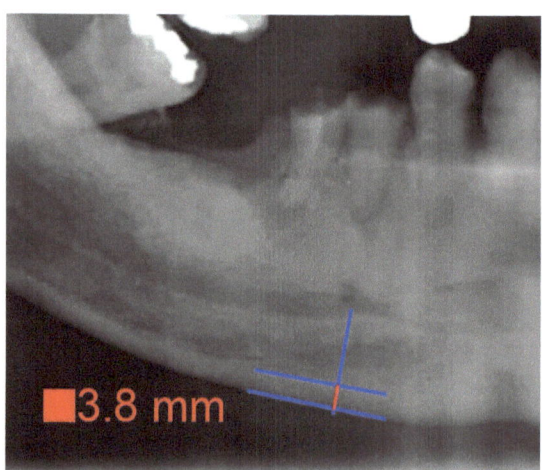

Figure 2-3. *Panoramic radiographic measurement of the width of the inferior mandibular cortex (MCW index).*

Imaging assessment of alveolar bone quality

Lekholm and Zarb (1985) classification[18]

The most commonly used radiographic classification of alveolar bone in dental implant researches was established by Lekholm and Zarb (1985).[18] This classification also takes into consideration the surgeon's tactile perception during drilling of implant site and implant placement. Alveolar bone tissue is classified into different categories, based on observations performed on radiographic images. This classification was described as inaccurate for predicting the insertion torque,[19] as it is subjective, and depends on the opinion of the professional.[20] According to this classification, the quality of alveolar bone is divided into four categories:

Q1 = residual bone formed by homogeneous cortical bone.
Q2 = residual bone formed by a thick layer of cortical bone surrounding dense trabecular bone.
Q3 = residual bone formed by a thin layer of cortical bone surrounding dense trabecular bone.
Q4 = residual bone formed by a thin layer of cortical bone surrounding low-density trabecular bone.

There is a controversy in the literature regarding the use of Lekholm and Zarb (1985) classification. Despite the fact that the original description of the classification takes into account the surgeon's tactile perception, several previous studies used this classification taking only 2D radiographic findings into consideration.[21-23] Other studies used CT images to define the different categories, thus developing new classifications.[24,25] Only a few studies actually considered the original features of the classification.[26,27]

University of California - Los Angeles (UCLA) classification[28]

Researchers from UCLA presented a classification of edentulous alveolar bone according to bone volume and shape, as assessed in 3D radiographic images. The bone volume in the horizontal and vertical dimensions was assessed by clinical observations during placement of implants in the ideal restorative driven positions. Eight different classes were defined according to the degree of deficient ridge volume, taking into consideration both vertical and horizontal planes.[28]

Class I (a): No deficiency in the horizontal or vertical dimension for placement of dental implant in the optimal restoratively driven position.
Class II minor (b): Alveolar crest with minor horizontal deficiency, but no horizontal deficiency at the apical level.
Class II major (c): Alveolar crest with major horizontal deficiency, but no horizontal deficiency at the apical level.
Class III minor (d): Alveolar crest with no horizontal deficiency, but minor horizontal deficiency at the apical level.
Class III major (e): Alveolar crest with no horizontal deficiency, but major horizontal deficiency at the apical level.
Class IV (f): Horizontal deficiency at both crestal and apical levels, but still with adequate vertical bone.
Class V (g): Lack of vertical bone but still with adequate horizontal dimensions.
Class VI (h): Insufficient bone in both vertical and horizontal dimensions (horizontal deficiency can be at the crest and/or apical levels).

The above-mentioned classification was also used as a base of further developed classifications, such as the one described by S. Iida.[29]

Modified UCLA alveolar bone classification by S. Iida[29]

By using the UCLA edentulous alveolar ridge classification as a reference, a group of authors developed a new radiographic classification for alveolar bone of implant sites.[29] Categories were divided as following:

Type I: Sufficient alveolar shape for placement of implants (a + b).
Type II: Insufficient amount of bone on the buccal side (d + e).
Type III: Alveolar crest with knife-edge shape but sufficient bone height (c + f).
Type IV: The alveolar bone height of the ridge is insufficient for implant placement (g + h).

Alveolar bone classifications based on CT images using Hounsfield Units

A study by Norton and Gamble (2001)[24] addressed the relationship between alveolar bone mineral density bone and the subjective classification previously described by Lekholm and Zarb (1985).[18] The new bone quality classification proposed is therefore based on bone density (HU) as following:

Q1: more than 850 HU.
Q2-Q3: 500–850.
Q4: 0–500 HU.
Any additional category: less than 0 HU.

According to the findings of the mentioned study, it was not possible to set boundary values between Q2 and Q3 categories.[24] Furthermore, bone density measurements (HU) of this study were obtained from the whole implant insertion site. As a result, the cortical layer of the ridge was also included in the region of interest measured. This is one of the ways to perform gray-scale analysis of dental implant sites although it differs from a similar study that also suggested another radiographic classification for alveolar bone.

In contrast with the above-mentioned classification, a study by de Oliveira and collaborators[25] introduced a radiographic classification based only on findings of trabecular bone density. The three categories of trabecular bone were divided as following:

Q1: more than 400 HU.
Q2-Q3: 200–400 HU.
Q4: less than 200 HU.

Alveolar bone assessment on CBCT images

There is agreement among authors of different studies regarding the importance of diagnostic imaging of the alveolar bone for planning implant surgeries. Among the main diagnostic applications of CT for oral implantology is the gray-scale analysis with pixel values. While this analysis has been widely described using the Hounsfield scale developed for spiral CT,[24,25,30] various laboratory and clinical studies also validated CBCT for quantitative analysis of bone tissue of the ridge.[31-33] It was observed a significant correlation between pixel values taken from CBCT images of dental implant sites and the results of morphometric analysis of bone specimens retrieved from the respective sites.[31,34,35] However, only one recent study assessed the specificity and sensitivity of gray-scale analysis for the diagnosis of implant placement surgeries.[35]

Besides the use of pixel values, it is also possible to use HU to quantify gray-scale measurements performed on CBCT images. For this purpose, it is necessary to use attenuation and calibration coefficients prior to carrying out the scans. One previous study addressed this issue and proposed a derivation of the Hounsfield scale for use in CBCT images.[36]

What is the Hounsfield Scale?

The Hounsfield scale is a quantitative measurement of radiodensity in a linear scale of gray shades expressed in HU. It involves a quantitative transformation of the x-ray attenuation coefficient. The arbitrary scale is defined by water, which has a value of 0 HU, and air, with a value of -1000 HU.

Aranyarachkul and collaborators[37] compared bone density measurements with HU from spiral CT and CBCT. It was observed that the pixel values of CBCT were generally higher than the corresponding values of spiral CT. Parametric correlation between the pixel values of both techniques was significantly strong, as demonstrated by Pearson correlation coefficients ranging from 0.92 to 0.98. Similarly, the use of HU for CBCT was also indicated as a potential diagnostic tool for bone tissue changes.[38,39]

Among the existing findings from association studies, it was observed that the radiographic bone density of implant sites obtained with CBCT (Figure 2-4) and implant insertion torque had significant correlation in animal experiments,[32] and human alveolar bone samples.[33] However, another article found no significant correlation for CBCT region of interests (ROI) taken from posterior implant sites.[39] To address the aforementioned controversy, a clinical and radiographic alveolar bone classification was developed to predict insertion torque of dental implant.[35]

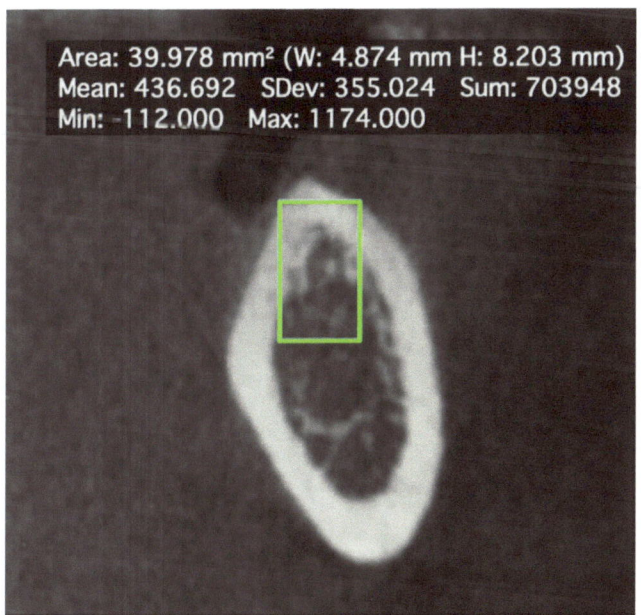

Figure 2-4. *Pixel values of a rectangular ROI (OsiriX) delimited in a CBCT slice of an implant site in posterior mandible.*

Radiographic classification for prediction of insertion torque of dental implants.[35]

Recently, Tamimi and Cortes[35] developed a new clinical and radiographic classification for prediction of insertion torque. In their study, images from panoramic radiographs and CBCT scans, as well as micro-CT and histological findings from bone samples of the implant sites were taken into consideration.

Insertion torque is influenced by bone quality and quantity, type of implant design and surgical technique.[5,7,8] In the new classification study,[35] a single surgeon performed all procedures using the same type and dimensions of implants. As a result, since the other factors were fixed, the authors were able to evaluate the solely influence of alveolar bone features on implant insertion torque.[35]

In their study,[35] multiple variables quantifying trabecular bone (i.e. radiographic bone density using gray-scale analysis; bone volume per total volume (BV/TV) using both micro-CT and histology) were assessed. All of them presented either none or poor correlations with the peak insertion torque. On the other hand, most methods assessing cortical bone (DXA, MCI and ridge cortical thickness) presented significant strong correlations with the peak insertion torque.[35] These findings support a histomorphometric study that found no significant correlation between histomorphometric analysis of BV/TV and peak insertion torque,[40] and another study concluding that the amount of cortical bone in contact with the implant is proportional to its insertion torque.[41] Moreover, the quantitative results presented[35] confirm the evidences of the influence of alveolar cortical layer on the tactile resistance experienced by the surgeon during drilling and on implant stability, as described by previous studies using subjective bone classifications.[3,18]

Despite the above-mentioned statistical results, no significant correlation between radiographic bone density taken from CBCT and peak insertion torque was found.[35] This finding is in agreement with a previous study.[39] In contrast, another study found a strong correlation between radiographic bone density and peak insertion torque.[33] However, the aforementioned study included a higher number of maxillary implant sites. As a result, the role of the cortical layer in providing high insertion torques could not be entirely addressed.

Despite the absence of correlation between pixel values and torque, the new classification study[35] also found that radiographic bone density from pre-operative CBCT scans (taken with the i-CAT Classic® device) presents strong significant correlations with BV/TV values obtained from both μ-CT and histology, as observed by a previous study.[31] This observation, however, has not been confirmed in postoperative CBCT,[42] which seems to indicate that beam-hardening artifacts caused by implant metallic bodies could be altering radiographic bone density results.

Panoramic radiographs have also an important value in the classification proposed by Tamimi and Cortes.[35] In addition, their study was the first to address the correlation of panoramic radiographic indices with peak insertion torque. Mandibular cortical index presented a weak to moderate inverse correlation with torque (r=-0.373, p=0.039). However, this variable was found to be strongly associated with peak insertion torque outcomes, according to the adjusted odds ratio analysis (AOR=13.32, 95% CI=1.32-134.47). Despite the fact that MCI is a radiographic indicator for systemic bone quality,[17] it has also been found to play an important role in the diagnostic performance of the classification to predict implant insertion torque, according to the sensitivity and specificity analyses presented by the authors.[35] Furthermore, the correlation between MCI and MCW and patients' age observed in their study supports results from articles that validated these indices to predict systemic bone alterations such as osteoporosis, since systemic bone density is expected to decrease as the patient grow older.[12]

Sensitivity and specificity are useful diagnostic performance analyses, and are adequate to assess prediction of insertion torque. In addition, this is the first objective radiographic classification developed to predict high insertion torque of implants, using digital panoramic radiographs, commonly used for general screening at first patient attendance,[43] and pre-operative CBCT, in accordance with ALARA radiation safety guidelines.[44] The classification[35] was based on MCI and ridge cortical thickness divided alveolar bone in 3 categories:

- Class I: when the inferior mandibular cortex has a normal appearance AND the ridge cortical layer at the alveolar crest is vertically thicker than 0.75mm.

- Class II: when either the inferior mandibular cortex has an eroded appearance OR the ridge cortical layer at the alveolar crest is vertically thinner than 0.75mm.
- Class III: when the inferior mandibular cortex has an eroded appearance AND the ridge cortical layer at the alveolar crest is vertically thinner than 0.75mm.

Implants placed in class I have 90% probability of having a high torque and could be planned for immediate loading. Similarly, implants placed in class III are predicted to have 100% probability of having a low torque. The authors state that such cases would require additional clinical measures to enhance the primary stability of implants, such as using tapered implant bodies or decreasing the diameter of the last drill. As a result, the new radiographic classification could be decisive for planning immediate loaded implants, and would also affect drilling sequence, and implant diameter and type selection.[35]

Implant insertion torque has been significantly correlated with survival rates of implants using immediate loading.[45] A study on single-tooth implants found that a torque greater than 32 Ncm is required to achieve osseointegration in cases of immediate loading.[46] Therefore, although the authors did not assess the impact of their radiographic classification on immediate loading, their data indicate that this classification could be useful to enhance treatment plan of such cases.[35]

The authors also state that, since success of immediate loading do not depend solely on insertion torque, future randomized clinical trials would be recommended to test the clinical application of their classification in patients receiving immediate loaded implants. Furthermore, although an appropriate sample size was achieved to test their hypothesis, the number of implants in each region of the jaws was low. Similarly, none of the implants were lost. As a result, the authors were not able to assess the impact of their classification on implant survival rates.[35] This issue could be addressed by future cohort studies with larger sample sizes and using different implant systems to evaluate the classification to predict implant insertion torque as a risk factor for implant loss in cases of immediate and conventional loading.

Morphometric and laboratorial diagnosis of the alveolar bone

In addition to the radiographic techniques used in the dental clinical practice, various quantitative and qualitative laboratory methods for assessing alveolar bone tissue have been described in the literature. Among them, the most used are histomorphometric analysis, micro-computed tomography and bone densitometry.

Bone histomorphometry was developed in the 1950s originally for the diagnosis of various metabolic bone diseases,[47-49] such as osteoporosis. As mentioned before, osteoporosis is recognized as loss of bone mineral density including deterioration of trabecular bone structure. Initially, some characteristics of trabecular bone such as high porosity and intricate orientation were observed at the macroscopic level. The microscopic technique was performed in two-dimensional slices (Figure 2-5), so that the trabecular structures could be measured by counting points and lines using optical microscopy or, more recently, by using technologic imaging analysis systems. Various mathematical formulas have been proposed to extrapolate 2D measurements to the third spatial dimension.[50] However, 3D trabecular measurements have been derived only from both area of measurement and trabecular perimeter, thus providing a limited description of the bone architecture.

On the other hand, histomorphometric analysis has been regarded as the gold standard technique for morphometric and structural assessment of bone tissue. The method is based on direct visualization of bone cells and their arrangement in the tissue using histological sections of a sample, thereby allowing for the diagnosis of alterations.[51] With this technique, several parameters can be evaluated with different histological staining methods. In studies on the osseointegration of dental implants and grafts, one of the most assessed parameters is the ratio of bone volume to the total volume of the bone sample (BV/TV).[40,52] Trabecular number can also be assessed as the number of trabeculae present in the field of the bone volume analyzed (Tb.N, mm-1). Trabecular thickness, in turn, can be calculated as the averaged thickness of the trabeculae present in the field of the bone volume analyzed (Tb.Th, µm).

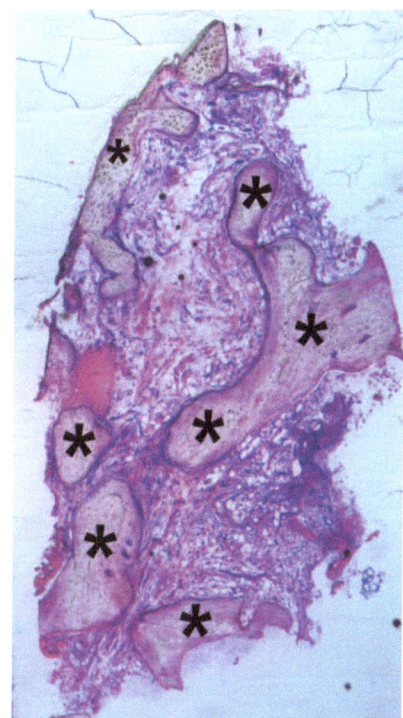

Figure 2-5. *Histological analysis of a bone sample retrieved from an implant site. Note the areas with bone tissue (asterisks).*

Another application of histomorphometry recently described in the literature is the evaluation and follow-up of socket healing after tooth extraction.[53]

Micro-computed tomography (micro-CT) is an x-ray technique similar to the ones of CT systems, but with much higher resolution (Figure 2-6). In this process, a number of two-dimensional radiographic images are stored while the bone sample and the set consisting of x-ray source and detector rotates.[54,55] During this procedure, internal tissue structures can be precisely reconstructed as a series of 2D cross-sections (up to 2600 in one scan), which will be then used to analyze morphological parameters in 2D and 3D. Similarly to histomorphometric analyses of alveolar bone tissue, BV/TV is also one of the most assessed parameters with micro-CT. However, unlike histomorphometric analysis, the evaluation process with micro-CT does not compromise the sample and does not require any special preparation for specimens. As a result, the imaging procedure with micro-CT is significantly faster. While CT images have an average size of pixel of 1 mm, micro-CT can acquire images with pixels of 0.7 micrometers.[51,54,55]

A wide range of clinical applications have been reported in the literature on micro-CT 3D analysis of bone tissue (Figure 2-7), including morphology, porosity and fractal analysis, as well as investigation of adjacent soft tissues.[41,51,54,55] Studies on bone morphometry found that the results from micro-CT are strongly correlated with those from histology and histomorphometry. Furthermore, micro-CT was also validated and described as a useful method for assessing the osseointegration of dental implants and bone grafts.[41,56]

Despite many studies have focused on the use of micro-CT for structural analysis of the trabecular bone, Particelli and collaborators[55] also tested the accuracy of micro-CT to analyze cortical bone. The aforementioned study included measurements such as the diameter of Haversian canals and the separation between them. There were no significant differences between micro-CT and conventional histomorphometric analysis. Furthermore, there were strong correlations between some numerical variables measured in both methods.

Bone densitometry with DXA has been considered the gold standard for measurements of systemic bone mineral density (BMD).[57] In addition, this method is also useful to assess local BMD of small bone tissue samples. Results of mandibular BMD analysis with densitometry were correlated with values of systemic bone mineral density obtained with lumbar bone densitometry.[58] However, local BMD analysis is not routinely available to the clinical professional, and standard measures have not yet been defined for the different regions of the alveolar ridge.

Bodic and collaborators[52] conducted a study on bone densitometry of tissue samples involving CT and micro-CT, and observed significant differences between density values obtained from symphysis, ramus and angle of the mandible. The densitometry results were not significantly correlated with CT and micro-CT, although the latter two were strongly correlated with each other. However, another study on patients undergoing hemodialysis treatment validated densitometry as an accurate method for evaluation of cortical bone.[59] According to the authors, femoral BMD results were strongly correlated with histological results for cortical porosity. In agreement with these results, another recent article addressed the correlation between BMD of small bone samples and their respective morphometric results.[35]

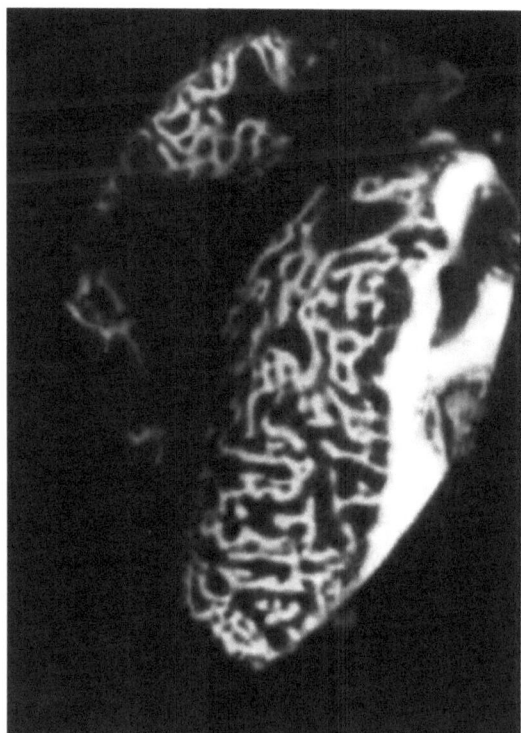

Figure 2-6. *2D micro-CT image used for morphometric analysis of bone sample retrieved from an implant site.*

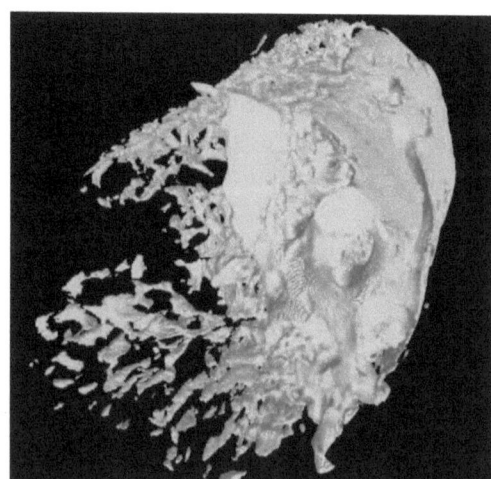

Figure 2-7. *3D reconstruction model of micro-CT used for morphometric analysis of bone sample retrieved from an implant site.*

Magnetic Resonance Imaging

Novel approaches to the application of magnetic resonance imaging (MRI) in dentistry have led to important advances in the field of oral diagnosis. Clinical MRI scans have proved useful in the assessment of the temporomandibular joint (TMJ),[60] caries lesions,[61] and sinus floor augmentation procedures.[62]

MRI provides 3D multiplanar imaging with satisfactory soft-tissue contrast using non-ionizing electromagnetic fields. MRI images are formed by radiofrequency signals that are generated from the spins of the nuclei of hydrogen (^{1}H) atoms.

In the bone tissue, hydrogen atoms can be found mainly in the water and protein contained in the bone matrix, and in the water and fat in marrow (Figures 2-8 and 2-9). This is because the total tissue volume of a bone mainly consists of the bone substance (i.e. extracellular calcified matrix) and the bone marrow that fills the porous spaces. With aging, the composition of bone marrow changes toward a higher number of fat tissue cells, and a higher bone marrow adipose volume, which is associated with age-related bone loss.

As a result, it is not possible to assess bone mineral content with conventional ^{1}H MRI. On the other hand, MRI images can also be obtained from the signal emitted by phosphorus (^{31}P) atoms present in the hydroxyapatite. This is a novel method named 31P solid-state magnetic resonance imaging (SMRI), which was developed to visualize bone mineral.[63] Nevertheless, this method cannot be performed in patients on clinical MRI scanners. Moreover, despite continuing research and many technological improvements, it is still challenging to achieve high contrast and high spatial resolution with MRI of solids.

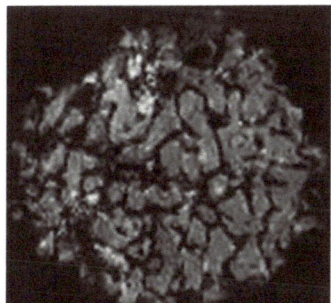

Figure 2-8. ^{1}H MRI of a bone sample obtained with a high-field device (14.56 Tesla).

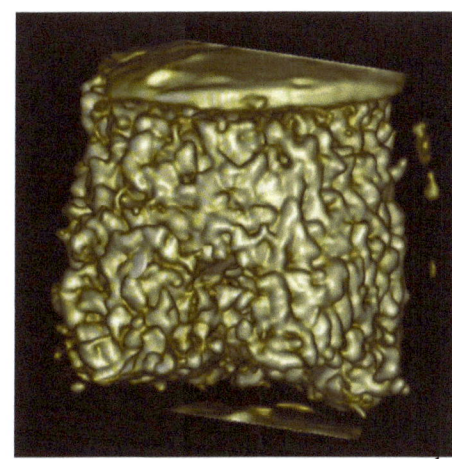

Figure 2-9. 3D reconstructed image from ^{1}H MRI of a bone sample obtained with a high-field device (14.56 Tesla).

Ultrasonography

One of the determinant factors affecting the healing process of a tissue is the blood supply. In this context, compromised vascularization may lead to alterations in bone remodeling capacity and integrity.[64] Furthermore, blood flow assessment is critical in defining the diagnosis of several important pathological conditions.

One method to assess blood supply is the Ultrasonography (US). This is a versatile, non-invasive and painless method of imaging diagnosis that does not also use ionizing radiation. It can also acquire sectional images of anatomic structures in any spatial orientation. In addition, US can be used in association with the Doppler effect, which enables assessing hemodynamics and includes dynamic features of both vascular architecture and blood flow in real time.[65]

A number of ultrasound applications have been described in the literature on oral diagnosis.[66-71] Applications include oral cancer diagnosis,[65] salivary gland imaging and assessment of mandibular vascularization. The latter is useful to detect blood flow changes in the inferior alveolar artery and its branches, as well as in the mental artery, which leaves the mandible through the mental foramen.

Another important clinical relevance is that the mental artery flow diminishes with age.[69,70] This condition has been described as a potential etiologic factor for alveolar bone atrophy.[69,72]

References

1. von Wowern N, Kollerup G. Symptomatic osteoporosis: a risk factor for residual ridge reduction of the jaws. J Prosthet Dent. 1992;67(5):656-60.

2. Jemt T, Lekholm U. Implant treatment in edentulous maxillae: a 5-year follow-up report on patients with different degrees of jaw resorption. Int J Oral Maxillofac Implants. 1995;10(3):303-11.

3. Misch CE. Bone classification, training keys to implant success. Dent Today. 1989;8(4):39-44.

4. Marco F, Milena F, Gianluca G, Vittoria O. Peri-implant osteogenesis in health and osteoporosis. Micron. 2005;36(7-8):630-44.

5. Meredith N. Assessment of implant stability as a prognostic determinant. Int J Prosthodont. 1998;11(5):491-501.

6. Trisi P, Perfetti G, Baldoni E, Berardi D, Colagiovanni M, Scogna G. Implant micromotion is related to peak insertion torque and bone density. Clin Oral Implants Res. 2009;20(5):467-71.

7. Javed F, Romanos GE. The role of primary stability for successful immediate loading of dental implants. A literature review. J Dent. 2010;38(8):612-20.

8. Marquezan M, Osorio A, Sant'Anna E, Souza MM, Maia L. Does bone mineral density influence the primary stability of dental implants? A systematic review. Clin Oral Implants Res. 2012;23(7):767-74.

9. Martinez H, Davarpanah M, Missika P, Celletti R, Lazzara R. Optimal implant stabilization in low density bone. Clin Oral Implants Res. 2001;12(5):423-32.

10. Scarfe WC, Farman AG, Sukovic P. Clinical applications of cone-beam computed tomography in dental practice. J Can Dent Assoc. 2006;72(1):75-80.

11. Cortes AR, Pinheiro LR, Umetsubo OS, Arita ES, Cavalcanti MG. Assessment of implant-related treatment with edited three-dimensional reconstructed images from cone-beam computed tomography: a technical note. J Oral Implantol. 2014;40(6):729-32

12. Taguchi A, Suei Y, Ohtsuka M, Otani K, Tanimoto K, Ohtaki M. Usefulness of panoramic radiography in the diagnosis of postmenopausal osteoporosis in women. Width and morphology of inferior cortex of the mandible. Dentomaxillofac Radiol. 1996;25(5):263-7.

13. Klemetti E, Kolmakov S, Heiskanen P, Vainio P, Lassila V. Panoramic mandibular index and bone mineral densities in postmenopausal women. Oral Surg Oral Med Oral Pathol. 1993;75(6):774-9.

14. Arita ES, Pippa MG, Marcucci M, Cardoso R, Cortes AR, Watanabe PC, et al. Assessment of osteoporotic alterations in achondroplastic patients: a case series. Clin Rheumatol. 2013;32(3):399-402.

15. Imirzalioglu P, Yuzugullu B, Gulsahi A. Correlation between residual ridge resorption and radiomorphometric indices. Gerodontology. 2012;29(2):e536-42.

16. Yuzugullu B, Gulsahi A, Imirzalioglu P. Radiomorphometric indices and their relation to alveolar bone loss in completely edentulous Turkish patients: a retrospective study. J Prosthet Dent. 2009;101(3):160-5.

17. Taguchi A, Sanada M, Krall E, Nakamoto T, Ohtsuka M, Suei Y, et al. Relationship between dental panoramic radiographic findings and biochemical markers of bone turnover. J Bone Miner Res. 2003;18(9):1689-94.

18. Lekholm U, Zarb G. Patient selection and preparation. Branemark, PI, Zarb, G & Albrektsson, T, eds Tissue-Integrated Prostheses: Osseointegration in Clinical Dentistry. Chicago: Quintessence; 1985. p. 233-40.

19. Friberg B, Sennerby L, Grondahl K, Bergstrom C, Back T, Lekholm U. On cutting torque measurements during implant placement: a 3-year clinical prospective study. Clin Implant Dent Relat Res. 1999;1(2):75-83.

20. Jeong KI, Kim SG, Oh JS, Jeong MA. Consideration of various bone quality evaluation methods. Implant Dent. 2013;22(1):55-9.

21. Molly L. Bone density and primary stability in implant therapy. Clin Oral Implants Res. 2006;17 Suppl 2:124-35.

22. Lindh C. Radiography of the mandible prior to endosseous implant treatment. Localization of the mandibular canal and assessment of trabecular bone. Swed Dent J Suppl. 1996;112:1-45.

23. Johansson B, Bäck T, Hirsch JM. Cutting torque measurements in conjunction with implant placement in grafted and nongrafted maxillas as an objective evaluation of bone density: a possible method for identifying early implant failures? Clin Implant Dent Relat Res 2004; 6:9-15.

24. Norton MR, Gamble C. Bone classification: an objective scale of bone density using the computerized tomography scan. Clin Oral Implants Res. 2001;12(1):79-84.

25. De Oliveira RC, Leles CR, Normanha LM, Lindh C, Ribeiro-Rotta RF. Assessments of trabecular bone density at implant sites on CT images. Oral Surg OralMed Oral Pathol Oral Radiol Endod 2008; 105:231-8.

26. Ribeiro-Rotta RF, De Oliveira RC, Dias DR, Lindh C, Leles CR. Bone tissue microarchitectural characteristics at
dental implant sites part 2: correlation with bone classification and primary stability. Clin Oral Implants Res 2014;
25:47-53.

27. Alsaadi G, Quirynen M, Michiels K, Jacobs R, Van Steenberghe D. A biomechanical assessment of the relation between the oral implant stability at insertion and subjective bone quality assessment. J Clin Periodontol 2007;34:359-66.

28. El-Ghareeb M, Moy PK, Aghaloo TL. The single-tooth dental implant: practical guidelines for hard tissue augmentation. J Calif Dent Assoc 2008;36: 869-84.

29. Wakimoto M, Matsumura T, Ueno T, Mizukawa N, Yanagi Y, Iida S. Bone quality and quantity of the anterior maxillary trabecular bone in dental implant sites. Clin Oral Impl Res 2012;23:1314-9.

30. Turkyilmaz I, Tumer C, Ozbek EN, Tozum TF. Relations between the bone density values from computerized tomography, and implant stability parameters: a clinical study of 230 regular platform implants. J Clin Periodontol. 2007;34(8):716-22.

31. Gonzalez-Garcia R, Monje F. The reliability of cone-beam computed tomography to assess bone density at dental implant recipient sites: a histomorphometric analysis by micro-CT. Clin Oral Implants Res. 2012 Aug;24(8):871-9.

32. Isoda K, Ayukawa Y, Tsukiyama Y, Sogo M, Matsushita Y, Koyano K. Relationship between the bone density estimated by cone-beam computed tomography and the primary stability of dental implants. Clin Oral Implants Res. 2012;23(7):832-6.

33. Salimov F, Tatli U, Kurkcu M, Akoglan M, Oztunc H, Kurtoglu C. Evaluation of relationship between preoperative bone density values derived from cone beam computed tomography and implant stability parameters: a clinical study. Clin Oral Implants Res. 2014;25:1016-21.

34. Monje A, Monje F, Gonzalez-Garcia R, Galindo-Moreno P, Rodriguez-Salvanes F, Wang HL. Comparison between microcomputed tomography and cone-beam computed tomography radiologic bone to assess atrophic posterior maxilla density and microarchitecture. Clin Oral Implants Res. 2014;25(6):723-8.

35. Cortes AR, Eimar H, Barbosa JS, Costa C, Arita ES, Tamimi F. Sensitivity and specificity of radiographic methods for predicting insertion torque of dental implants. Journal of Periodontology 2015;86:646-55.

36. Mah P, Reeves TE, McDavid WD. Deriving Hounsfield units using grey levels in cone beam computed tomography. Dentomaxillofac Radiol. 2010;39(6):323-35.

37. Aranyarachkul P, Caruso J, Gantes B, Schulz E, Riggs M, Dus I, et al. Bone density assessments of dental implant sites: 2. Quantitative cone-beam computerized tomography. Int J Oral Maxillofac Implants. 2005;20(3):416-24.

38. Cankaya AB, Erdem MA, Isler SC, Demircan S, Soluk M, Kasapoglu C, et al. Use of cone-beam computerized tomography for evaluation of bisphosphonate-associated osteonecrosis of the jaws in an experimental rat model. Int J Med Sci. 2011;8(8):667-72.

39. Fuster-Torres MA, Penarrocha-Diago M, Penarrocha-Oltra D. Relationships between bone density values from cone beam computed tomography, maximum insertion torque, and resonance frequency analysis at implant placement: a pilot study. Int J Oral Maxillofac Implants. 2011;26(5):1051-6.

40. Nkenke E, Hahn M, Weinzierl K, Radespiel-Troger M, Neukam FW, Engelke K. Implant stability and histomorphometry: a correlation study in human cadavers using stepped cylinder implants. Clin Oral Implants Res. 2003;14(5):601-9.

41. Hsu JT, Huang HL, Chang CH, Tsai MT, Hung WC, Fuh LJ. Relationship of three-dimensional bone-to-implant contact to primary implant stability and peri-implant bone strain in immediate loading: microcomputed tomographic and in vitro analyses. Int J Oral Maxillofac Implants. 2013;28(2):367-74.

42. Corpas Ldos S, Jacobs R, Quirynen M, Huang Y, Naert I, Duyck J. Peri-implant bone tissue assessment by comparing the outcome of intra-oral radiograph and cone beam computed tomography analyses to the histological standard. Clin Oral Implants Res. 2011;22(5):492-9.

43. Rushton VE, Horner K, Worthington HV. Factors influencing the selection of panoramic radiography in general dental practice. J Dent. 1999;27(8):565-71.

44. Dykstra BA. ALARA and radiation in the dental office: current state of affair. Dent Today. 2011;30(3):14, 6, 8.

45. Cannizzaro G, Leone M, Ferri V, Viola P, Gelpi F, Esposito M. Immediate loading of single implants inserted flapless with medium or high insertion torque: a 6-month follow-up of a split-mouth randomised controlled trial. Eur J Oral Implantol. 2012;5:333-42.

46. Ottoni JM, Oliveira ZF, Mansini R, Cabral AM. Correlation between placement torque and survival of single-tooth implants. Int J Oral Maxillofac Implants. 2005;20:769-76.

47. Villanueva AR, Jaworski ZF, Hitt O, Sarnsethsiri P, Frost HM. Cellular-level bone resorption in chronic renal failure and primary hyperparathyroidism. A tetracycline-based evaluation. Calcif Tissue Res. 1970;5(4):288-304.

48. Meunier P, Aaron J, Edouard C, Vignon G. Osteoporosis and the replacement of cell populations of the marrow by adipose tissue. A quantitative study of 84 iliac bone biopsies. Clin Orthop Relat Res. 1971;80:147-54.

49. Frost HM. Does bone mass equate with bone health? An argument for the negative. J Clin Densitom. 2001;4(3):179-84.

50. Parfitt AM, Drezner MK, Glorieux FH, Kanis JA, Malluche H, Meunier PJ, et al. Bone histomorphometry: standardization of nomenclature, symbols, and units. Report of the ASBMR Histomorphometry Nomenclature Committee. J Bone Miner Res. 1987;2(6):595-610.

51. Chappard D, Retailleau-Gaborit N, Legrand E, Basle MF, Audran M. Comparison insight bone measurements by histomorphometry and microCT. J Bone Miner Res. 2005;20(7):1177-84.

52. Bodic F, Amouriq Y, Gayet-Delacroix M, Maugars Y, Hamel L, Basle MF, et al. Relationships between bone mass and micro-architecture at the mandible and iliac bone in edentulous subjects: a dual X-ray absorptiometry, computerised tomography and microcomputed tomography study. Gerodontology. 2012;29(2):e585-94.

53. Clozza E, Pea M, Cavalli F, Moimas L, Di Lenarda R, Biasotto M. Healing of fresh extraction sockets filled with bioactive glass particles: histological findings in humans. Clin Implant Dent Relat Res. 2014;16(1):145-53.

54. Feldkamp LA, Goldstein SA, Parfitt AM, Jesion G, Kleerekoper M. The direct examination of three-dimensional bone architecture in vitro by computed tomography. J Bone Miner Res. 1989;4(1):3-11.

55. Particelli F, Mecozzi L, Beraudi A, Montesi M, Baruffaldi F, Viceconti M. A comparison between micro-CT and histology for the evaluation of cortical bone: effect of polymethylmethacrylate embedding on structural parameters. J Microsc. 2012;245(3):302-10.

56. Huang HL, Chen MY, Hsu JT, Li YF, Chang CH, Chen KT. Three-dimensional bone structure and bone mineral density evaluations of autogenous bone graft after sinus augmentation: a microcomputed tomography analysis. Clin Oral Implants Res. 2012;23(9):1098-103.

57. Devlin J, Lilley J, Gough A, Huissoon A, Holder R, Reece R, et al. Clinical associations of dual-energy X-ray absorptiometry measurement of hand bone mass in rheumatoid arthritis. Br J Rheumatol. 1996;35(12):1256-62.

58. Horner K, Devlin H, Alsop CW, Hodgkinson IM, Adams JE. Mandibular bone mineral density as a predictor of skeletal osteoporosis. Br J Radiol. 1996;69(827):1019-2.

59. Adragao T, Herberth J, Monier-Faugere MC, Branscum AJ, Ferreira A, Frazao JM, et al. Femoral bone mineral density reflects histologically determined cortical bone volume in hemodialysis patients. Osteoporos Int. 2010;21(4):619-25.

60. Nagamatsu-Sakaguchi C, Maekawa K, Ono T, et al. Test-retest reliability of MRI-based disk position diagnosis of the temporomandibular joint. Clin Oral Investig. 2012;16:101-8.

61. Bracher AK, Hofmann C, Bornstedt A, et al. Ultrashort echo time (UTE) MRI for the assessment of caries lesions. Dentomaxillofac Radiol. 2013;42:20120321.

62. Senel FC, Duran S, Icten O, Izbudak I, Cizmeci F. Assessment of the sinus lift operation by magnetic resonance imaging. Br J Oral Maxillofac Surg. 2006;44:511-4.

63. Wu Y, Reese TG, Cao H, Hrovat MI, Toddes SP, Lemdiasov RA, Ackerman JL. Bone mineral imaged in vivo by 31P solid state MRI of human wrists. J Magn Reson Imaging. 2011;34(3):623-33.

64. McGregor AD, MacDonald DG. Post-irradiation changes in the blood vessels of the adult human mandible. Br J Oral Maxillofac Surg. 1995;33:15-28.

65. Kagawa T, Yuasa K, Fukunari F, Shiraishi T, Miwa K. Quantitative evaluation of vascularity within cervical lymph nodes using Doppler ultrasound in patients with oral cancer: relation to lymph node size. Dentomaxillofac Radiol. 2011;40:415-21.

66. Jones JK, Frost DE. Ultrasound as a diagnostic aid in maxillofacial surgery. Report of a case. Oral Surg Oral Med Oral Pathol. 1984;57:589-94.

67. Bavitz JB, Harn SD, Homze EJ. Arterial supply to the floor of the mouth and lingual gingiva. Oral Surg Oral Med Oral Pathol. 1994;77:232-5.

68. Carotti M, Salaffi F, Manganelli P, Argalia G. Ultrasonography and colour doppler sonography of salivary glands in primary Sjogren's syndrome. Clin Rheumatol. 2001;20:213-9.

69. Eiseman B, Johnson LR, Coll JR. Ultrasound measurement of mandibular arterial blood supply: techniques for defining ischemia in the pathogenesis of alveolar ridge atrophy and tooth loss in the elderly? J Oral Maxillofac Surg. 2005;63:28-35.

70. Klein MO, Grotz KA, Manefeld B, Kann PH, Al-Nawas B. Ultrasound transmission velocity for noninvasive evaluation of jaw bone quality in vivo before dental implantation. Ultrasound Med Biol. 2008;34:1966-71.

71. Lustig JP, London D, Dor BL, Yanko R. Ultrasound identification and quantitative measurement of blood supply to the anterior part of the mandible. Oral Surg Oral Med Oral Pathol Oral Radiol Endod. 2003;96:625-9.

72. Baladi MG, Tucunduva Neto RCM, Cortes AR, Aoki EM, Arita ES, Freitas CF. Ultrasound analysis of mental artery flow in elderly patients: a case–control study. Dentomaxillofac Radiol 2015; 44: 20150097

CHAPTER 3

IMAGE-GUIDED IMPLANT SURGERY

Jorge de Sá Barbosa

José Marcio Barbosa Leite do Amaral

Arthur Rodriguez Gonzalez Cortes

History

In the past decades, implant surgical planning was basically determined by the remaining alveolar bone availability. Surgical plans were usually based on clinical findings combined with the analysis of two-dimensional images with minimal concern regarding the final aspect of the prosthesis to be supported by the implants.[1] Several studies showed that this philosophy could prevent important achievements of oral rehabilitations, such as an ideal occlusal pattern, adequate masticatory function, prosthesis aesthetics, and therefore decreasing the longevity of the clinical results.[2-4]

With the advent of surgical guides made using diagnostic wax-up on study casts, clinical outcomes of implant treatments started to be improved. In this context, CBCT with 3D features was validated as the standard radiographic examination for planning implant placements.[5] For many years, however, the above-mentioned tools have been used without any connection between then, providing limited results from implant placement surgeries. The first clinical tool obtained from the 3D CBCT images that were loaded into implant planning softwares was the rapid prototyping model from CAD/CAM technology. This has been widely applied in oral implantology for the fabrication of precise surgical templates (Figure 3-1) produced by stereolithography (i.e. polymer copies of anatomical structures to be considered during the surgical procedure) (Figure 3-2). Stereolithographic surgical guides derived from CBCT images have been regarded as useful tools to ensure correct

execution of a virtual surgical plan. Therefore, this technology allows the dentist to plan and perform surgery on a three-dimensional copy of the patient's bone structure (Figure 3-3). It is also possible to simulate implant placement and produce prosthetic guides based on the optimal implant positions (Figure 3-4A). This technique leads to safer surgical procedures (Figure 3-4B) and faster treatment times,[6,7] as well as more predictable results (Figure 3-4C).

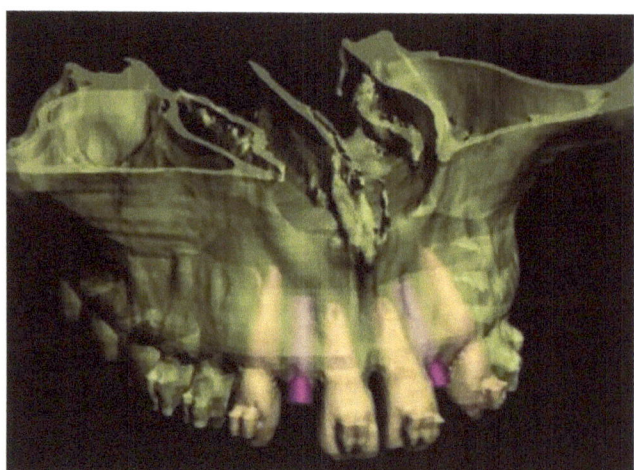

Figure 3-1. *3D reconstructed image of a virtual implant planning.*

There is ongoing research on the interactivity between 3D CBCT imaging features and rapid prototyping models. New software interfaces have been created and enhanced with the increasing focus of researches on the integration of CAD systems (Computer Aided Design) and CAM (Computer Aided Manufacturing).[8,9]

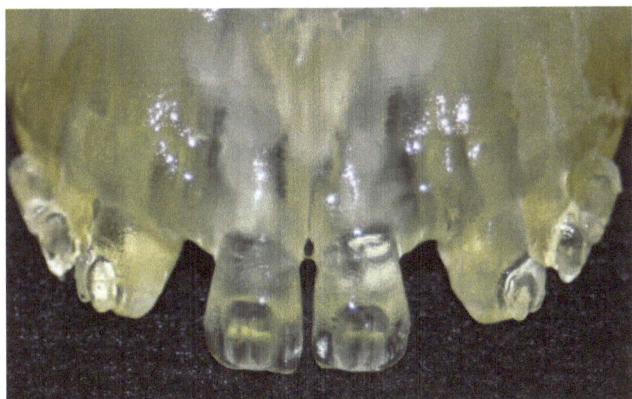

Figure 3-2. *Rapid prototyping model made from the virtual implant planning shown in Figure 3-1*

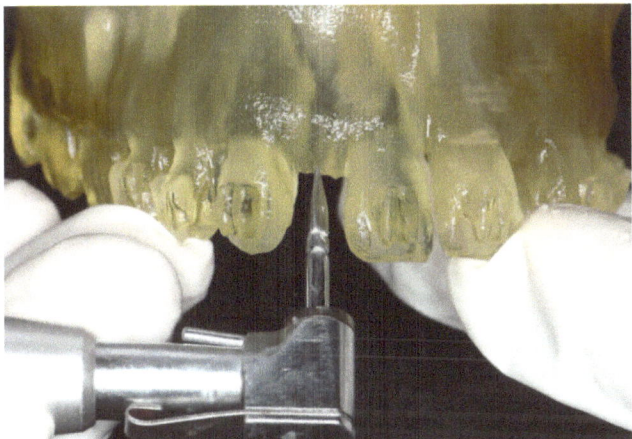

Figure 3-3. *Implant surgery simulation.*

Virtual implant planning

As briefly mentioned in the chapter 1, the virtual surgical planning consists in evaluating important anatomical landmarks and bone availability by using a CBCT imaging software with 3D interactivity, and performing measurements and implant placement simulations. Currently, the aforementioned tasks can be accomplished with the use of either DICOM (Digital Imaging and Communications in Medicine) viewers dedicated for radiology, or implant planning softwares. Some of the DICOM viewers are developed by manufacturers of CBCT devices and may also have implant planning tools.[10,11]

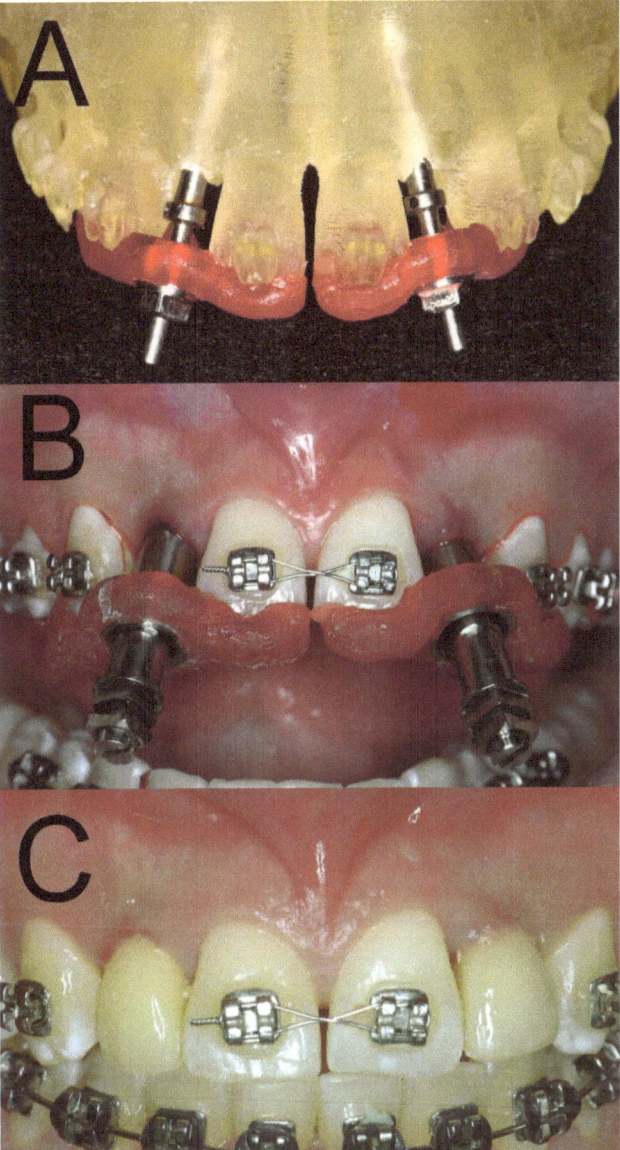

Figure 3-4. *Oral rehabilitation with image-guided surgery. A) Surgical guide development with acrylic resin. B) Flapless surgery performed to place the implants with the surgical guide. C) Immediate prosthesis installed.*

Despite the higher number of 3D features provided by DICOM viewers, implant planning softwares are the most used to generate and visualize stereolithographic surgical guides derived from CBCT images. There is an increasing focus of researches on the comparison between these two types of softwares. Small significant differences in accuracy of measurements have been reported between different softwares. This could directly affect the accuracy of implant placement.[12,13]

Virtual implant planning features:
- Assessment of anatomical landmarks
- Linear measurements of the alveolar bone height and width
- Estimation of bone density by using gray-scale analysis with pixel values
- Selection of type, size and number of implants
- Selection and refinement of implant position and inclination in multiple planes
- Assessment of the characteristics of the final prosthesis and its spatial relationship with the implants
- Visualization of the surgical guide
- Selection of optimal locations for the fixation screws of the surgical guide
- Exportation of the entire dataset to generate the stereolithographic surgical guide

Image-Guided surgery

The first requirement to plan and perform an image-guided surgery is to establish a logical sequence between rehabilitation prosthetic plan and implant placement surgical plan.[14,15] Therefore, the virtual surgical plan and the derived stereolithographic surgical guide should be based on a prosthetic plan, in order to promote a greater predictability of the results of the oral rehabilitation. The main benefits of implant surgeries that are guided by CT images are decreased surgical trauma and less short-term postoperative discomfort, which may be attributed to the use of a flapless approach. This technique allows maintaining the periosteum and blood supply to the alveolar bone tissue, leading to decreased contamination and surgical time.[19] These features, in turn, increase the predictability of clinical outcomes of immediate loading cases.

Currently, there are a number of guided surgery systems. One of the reasons is that most of the dental implant and software manufacturers have created their own system, as a result of the growing technological demand in the field of oral surgery. Systems of commercial brands differ in a number of factors, such as software 3D features, drill and implant dimensions, and number of dental implants recommended for full-arch rehabilitations.

Guided surgery is indicated for total or partial rehabilitation of the jaws. A larger volume of remaining bone available at the ridge facilitates the procedure. However, alveolar ridge atrophy has been described as a factor that does not prevent the professional from performing an image-guided surgery.[16] Basically, image-guided surgery allows the professional to transfer the exact implant positions that were virtually planned to the patient's mouth (Figure 3-5).[17]

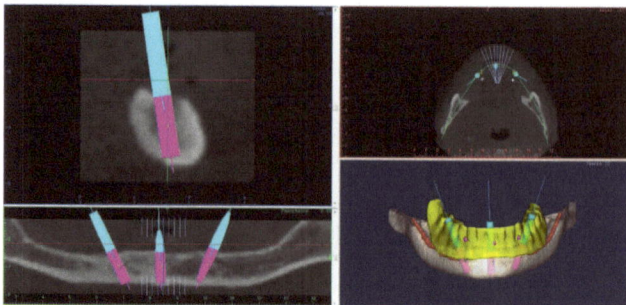

Figure 3-5. *Virtual implant planning with the DentalSlice® software (Bioparts, São Paulo, Brazil).*

Stereolithographic surgical guides
The prototyped models and surgical guides for oral implantology are made using CAD/CAM technology with laser sintering. In this process, each layer of liquid polymer is deposited and cured gradually by laser.[18,19] The entire process is precisely controlled by computers. These layers are superimposed and polymerized until the anatomical model or surgical guide is generated. The initial data come from a CBCT dataset and are processed on the computer to produce the prototyping model. Its accuracy depends on the quality of the CBCT acquisition protocol and image processing. It has been concluded that most anatomical models show dimensional stability with variations up to 0.6 milimeters.[20]

For the production of a surgical guide (Figure 3-6), it is required that the prosthetic rehabilitation plan is previously developed in order to design the guide. In this case, a double scanning procedure can be performed. The first scan acquires images of the patient with the tomographic guide in position. The tomographic guide is based on the design of a duplicate of an existing prosthesis marked with hyperdense materials (e.g. gutta-percha). The second scan is performed to acquire images of the tomographic guide alone. The rationale of using marks of hyperdense materials is to combine the images of the patient and of the tomographic guide.

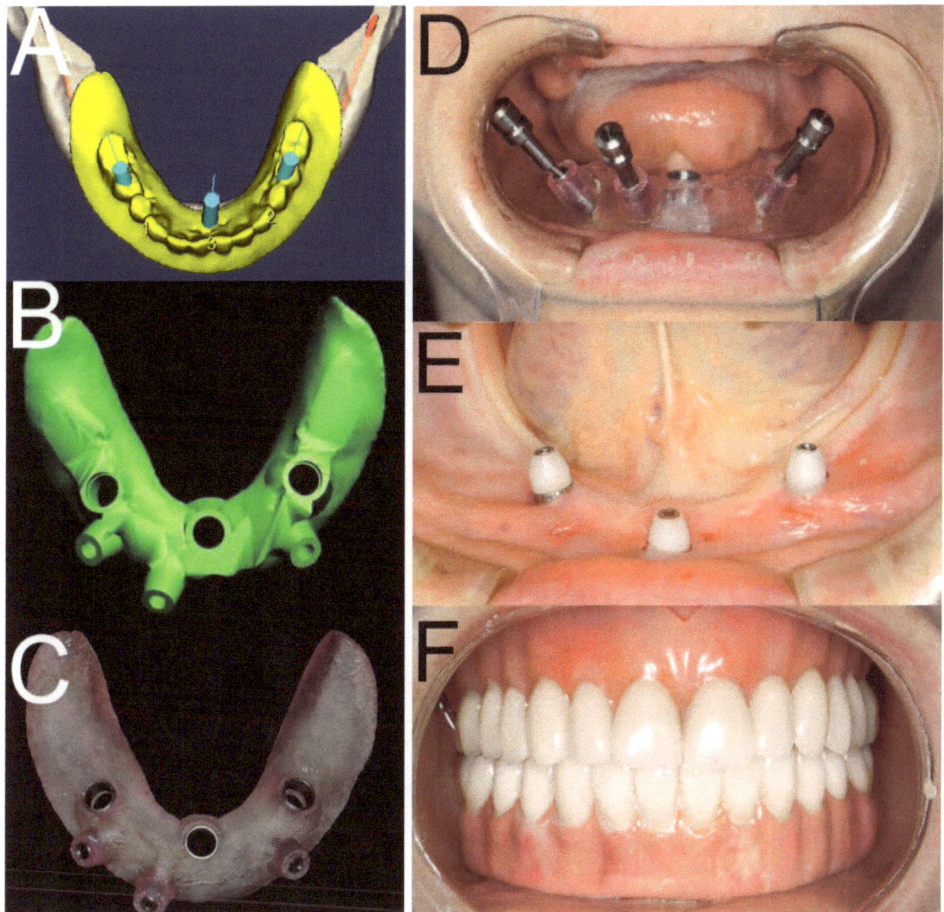

Figure 3-6. *Clinical application of the surgical guide generated from the virtual implant planning shown in Figure 3-5. A) 3D CBCT images of implant positions. B) Digital design. C) Manufactured surgical guide. D) Surgical guide in position. E) Implants with prosthetic abutments. F) Final prosthetic result.*

As a result, the professional is able to plan the implants while viewing their spatial relationship with the prosthesis to be installed in the patient. After choosing optimal positions, the virtual plan is finally exported to produce the stereolithographic surgical guide, which will have drilling sleeves that fits the drill diameter of the corresponding implant system. Surgical guides can be supported by soft tissues, by bone, or by remaining teeth (in case of partial restorations). To achieve bone support, the surgical guide is fixed to the alveolar bone with small stabilizing screws.

The precision of implant surgeries performed with stereolithographic surgical guides (Figure 3-7) has been assessed by some studies comparing implant positions defined in virtual planning with the actual positions of the implants assessed after surgical placement.[16,19,21,22,24] These studies found significant differences, such as mean deviations ranging from 0.2 mm in the coronal plane with 1.1 degrees of angular discrepancy to 1.5 mm in the

coronal plane with values around seven degrees of angular discrepancy. Intraoperative complications in cases using stereolithographic surgical guides are usually related to excessive drilling deviation, generally caused by factors such as small mouth opening, lack of experience of the surgeon and quality of the surgical guide used, which may be compromised if the guide is not stable during drilling.[25]

Benefits to patients undergoing image-guided surgery:
- Less postoperative pain
- Easy to understand the procedure
- Faster treatment times
- Low rates of surgical complication
- Good patient satisfaction

The process of using guides for stereolithography is typically based on a protocol consisting of:

1- Rehabilitation planning with diagnostic wax-up, preparation of the future prosthesis design and prosthesis duplication (tomographic guide)
2- Tomographic guide marking with hyperdense material (usually gutta-percha)
3- Computed tomographic dual scanning (i.e. a first acquisition of patient images with the tomographic guide in position, usually with a heavy silicone impression to stabilize the guide, and a second acquisition of the tomographic guide alone.
4- Virtual implant planning in specific software with the images of the final prosthesis design overlapping anatomical structures.
5- Exporting and sending the files to the company that will manufacture of the surgical guide.
6- Flapless implant surgery with surgical guide.
7- Rehabilitation with immediate provisional or final prosthesis

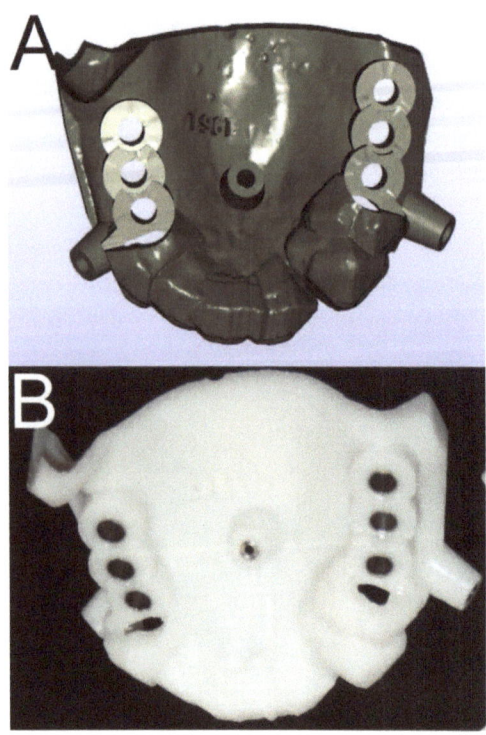

Figure 3-7. *Stereolithographic surgical guide. A) 3D image. B) Manufactured guide (Bioparts, São Paulo, Brazil).*

Chairside milled surgical guides
Basically following the same principles of guides generated by stereolithography, milled surgical

guides are indicated for partial rehabilitations and can be generated at the chairside. The professional can monitor the whole process, thus reducing its cost and time.[26] Patients' anatomical information can be obtained using either an intraoral scanner, or by scanning dental study casts. Intraoral scanners have advantages such as no discomfort caused by impression materials and faster procedure times. Bone and soft tissue images can be displayed together with surgical and prosthetic planning. This method can also be used for immediate loading.[27] The most common treatment procedure using chairside milled surgical guides follows some steps:

1- Rehabilitation planning with diagnostic wax-up and definition of the implant sites.
2- Guide production with thermoplastic material and adaptation of the CT markers provided by the manufacturer.
3- Computed tomographic scanning with CT guide in position usually with a heavy silicone impression to stabilize the guide.
4- Virtual prosthetic planning by CAD.
5- Virtual implant placement planning with images of prosthesis design overlapping anatomical structures.
6- Milling of the surgical guide by CAM.
7- Implant placement flapless surgery with surgical guide
8- Rehabilitation with immediate provisional or final prosthesis

With the technological evolution of the CAD/CAM system and intra-oral scanners, various systems are being produced to create interfaces between CT data and scanned intraoral images, eliminating the use of tomographic guides, and thus reducing costs and procedure time.[26,27]

Dynamic image-guided (navigation) surgery
Dynamic image-guided surgery was introduced a few years ago and pioneered in medical fields. It is a novel technique in the field of implant dentistry and offers a number of benefits. Like other techniques of image-guided surgery, it involves CT scanning.[28] Among the existing surgical navigation systems, optical tracking systems are the most commonly used. These systems include an infrared camera detector to track surgical instruments that are equipped with infrared light emitters. The position of the surgical instrument is continuously related to the

imaging data, thus providing the dynamic imaging navigation. Reference markers are used to establish a precise interface between the CT data and the actual surgical field. Those markers are placed in the surgical field and identified on the CT images. Another new technologic procedure is characterized by an initial intraoral laser scan used to fabricate a tracking array of standard sensors. The patient undergoes then a CT scan with this array placed in position. Virtual implant planning is performed in the specific software system.

In the case of dynamic image-guided surgery there is no drilling sleeves in the surgical guide. Instead, the guide will only send signals to provide information on the actual position of the drill in real time. This is done to compare surgical planning and execution, and if necessary, to make any required changes. The system also allows the professional to visualize images of the virtual prosthetic planning superimposing regular CT images of the patient to achieve optimal results in the rehabilitation. Some of the softwares are equipped with audible or visual signal that indicates drilling deviation from the planned position, or when there is proximity to any anatomical structures.

Some studies[28,29] have demonstrated osteotomy positions with less than one millimeter errors, as compared to the surgical planning, as well as high accuracy of the drilling angles. However, little is known regarding comparisons between the accuracy of surgical navigation and other methods of image-guided surgery. In this context, an *in vitro* study found more accurate results from implant surgeries performed with stereolithographic surgical guides.[30]

The use of surgical navigation has also been described for teaching purposes in other fields such as restorative dentistry. Future studies would be recommended to address more applications of this technology, which is increasingly present in the field of dentistry.[29]

References

1. Engelman MJ, Sorensen JA, Moy P. Optimum placement of osseointegrated implants. J Prosthet Dent 1988;59(4):467-73.

2. Rangert B, Krogh PH, Langer B, Van Roekel N. Bending overload and implant fracture: a retrospective clinical analysis. Int J Oral Maxillofacial Implants 1995;10 (3):326-34.

3. Hobkirk JA, Havthoulas TK. The influence of mandibular deformation, implant numbers, and loading position on detected forces in abutments supporting fixed implant superstructures. J Prosthet Dent 1998;80(2):169-74.

4. Stanford CM. Biomechanical and functional behavior of implants. Adv Dent Res 1999;13: 88-92.

5. Worthington P, Rubenstein J, Hatcher DC. The role of cone-beam computed tomography in the planning and placement of implants J Am Dent Assoc. 2010 ;141(3):19S-24S.

6- Sarment DP, Sukovic P, Clinthorne N. Accuracy of implant placement with a stereolithographic surgical guide. Int J Oral Maxillofacial Implants. 2003;18(4): 571-7.

7. Di Giacomo GA, Cury PR, Araujo NS, Sendyk WR, Sendyk CL. Clinical application of stereolithographic surgical guides for implant placement: preliminary results. J Periodontol 2005;76(4):503-7.

8. Ersoy AE, Türkyilmaz I, Ozan O, McGlumphy EA. Reliability of implant placement with stereolithographic surgical guides generated from computed tomography: clinical data from 94 implants. J Periodontol 2008 Aug; 79 (8): 1339-45.

9. Ozan O, I Türkyilmaz, Ersoy AE, McGlumphy EA, Rosenstiel SF.Clinical accuracy of 3 different types of computed tomography-derived stereolithographic surgical guides in implant placement. J Oral Maxillofacial Surg 2009; 67(2):394-401.

10. Maloney K, Bastidas J, Freeman K, Olson TR, Kraut RA. Cone beam computed tomography and simPlant materialize dental software versus direct measurement of the width and height of the posterior mandible: an anatomic study. J Oral Maxillofacial Surg 2011;69(7):1923-9.

11. Lund H, Gröndahl K, Gröndahl HG. Accuracy and precision of linear measurements in cone beam computed tomography Accuitomo® tomograms Obtained with different reconstruction techniques. Dentomaxillofac Radiol 2009;38(6):379-86.

12. Gaia BF, Pinheiro LR, Umetsubo OS, Costa FF, Cavalcanti MG. Comparison of precision and accuracy of linear measurements Performed by two different imaging software programs and Obtained from 3D CBCT images for Le Fort I osteotomy. Dentomaxillofac Radiol 2013;42(5):20,120,178.

13. dos Santos Jr O, Pinheiro LR, Umetsubo OS, Sales MA, Cavalcanti MG. Assessment of open

source software for CBCT in detecting mental additional foramina. Braz Oral Res 2013;27(2):128-35.

14. Varma DR. Free DICOM browsers. Indian J Radiol Imaging. 2008;18(1):12-16.

15. Beretta M, Poli PP, Maiorana C. Accuracy of computer-aided oral template-guided implant placement: a prospective clinical study. J Periodontal Implant Sci 2014;44(4):184-93.

16. Van Steenberghe D, Malevez C, Van Cleynenbreugel J, BouSerhal C, Dhoore A, Schutyser F et al. Accuracy of drilling guides for transfer is three-dimensional CT-based planning to placement of zygoma implants in human cadavers. Clin Oral Implants Res 2003;14:131-6.

17. Rubio-Serrano M, Albalat Estela S, Peñarrocha Diago M, Peñarrocha Diago M. Software applied to oral implantology: update. Med Oral Pathol Oral Cir Bucal 2008;13(10):E661-5.

18. Daas M, Assaf A, Given K, Makzoumé J. Computer-Guided Implant Surgery in Fresh Extraction Sockets and Immediate Loading of the Full Arch Restoration: A 2-Year Follow-Up Study of 14 Patients Treated consecutively. Int J Dent 2015;824:127.

19. Fortin T, Bosson JL, Coudert JL, Isidori M. Reliability of preoperative planning of an image-guided system for oral implant placement based on 3-dimensional images: An in vivo study. Int J Oral Maxillofacial Implants 2003;18:886-93.

20. Choi JY, Choi JH, Kim NK, Kim Y, Lee JK, Kim MK, Lee JH, Kim MJ. Analysis of errors in medical rapid prototyping models. Int J Oral Maxillofacial Surg. 2002;31(1):23-32.

21. Van Asshe N. Accuracy of implant placement based on presurgical planning of three dimensional cone-beam images: a pilot study. J Clin Periodontol 2007;34:816-21

22. Horwitz J, Zuabi O Machtei EE. Accuracy of the computerized tomography-guided template-assisted implant placement system: an in vitro study. Clin Oral Implants Res 2009;20:1156-62.

23. Sanna AM, Molly L., van Steenberghe D. Immediately loaded CAD-CAM manufactured fixed complete dentures using flapless implant placement procedures: a cohort study of consecutive patients. J Prosthet Dent. 2007;97(6):331-9

24. Vieira MD, Sotto-Maior BS, Barros CA, Reis ES, Francischone EC. Clinical accuracy of flapless computer-guided surgery for implant placement in edentulous arches. Int J Oral Maxillofacial Implants 2013;28(5):1347-51.

25. Abad-Gallegos M, Gómez-Santos L, Sánchez-Garcés MA, Piñera-Penalva M, Freixes-Gil J, Castro-García A, Gay-Escoda C. Complications of guided surgery and immediate loading in oral implantology: a report of 12 cases. Med Oral Pathol Oral Cir Bucal 2011;16(2):e220-4.

26. Bindl A. Clinical application of digital fully Cerec surgical guides made in-house. Int J Comput Dent. 2015; 18 (2): 163-75.

27. Reiz SD, Neugebauer J, Karapetian VE, L. Ritter Cerec meets Galileos - integrated implantology for virtual implant planning completely. Int J Comput Dent 2014;17(2):145-57.

28. Gaggl SG. Int J Oral Maxillofacial Implants. Assessment of accuracy of navigated implant placement in the maxilla. 2002;17(2):263-70.

29. Casap N, Wexler A, Persky N, Schneider, J. Lustmann Navigation surgery for dental implants: assessment of the accuracy of image guided implantology system. J Oral Maxillofacial Surg 2004;62(9 Suppl 2):116-9.

30. Kang HS, Lee JW, Lim HS, Kim YH, Kim MK. Verification of the usability of the navigation method in dental implant surgery: in vitro comparison with the stereolithographic surgical guide template method. Craniomaxillofac Surg 2014;42(7):1530-5.

CHAPTER 4

DENTAL IMPLANT FOLLOW-UP

Lucas Rodrigues Pinheiro
Arthur Rodriguez Gonzalez Cortes

Introduction

Partial and total rehabilitation of the edentulous jaws with titanium dental implants are well established as highly successful restorative therapies.[1-3] However, implants are susceptible to some complications. The most usual are perforation or injury of important anatomical structures, implant positioning error, peri-implant bone loss and fenestration of alveolar bone plates. Such complications may compromise stability, functionality or esthetics.[3,4] The detection of these complications can be challenging in some cases, for which radiographic imaging should be considered to assist in establishing a diagnosis.[5]

Two-dimensional radiographs are the most widely used techniques to monitor and diagnose bone loss (Figure 4-1). However, the images have limitations, such as geometric distortion, anatomic superimposition and inability to demonstrate buccal and lingual bone levels, resulting in low sensitivity for the detection of implant complications.[5-11]

Cone-beam computed tomography (CBCT) is now a readily available technique that provides volumetric acquisitions with relative low radiation doses. Multiplanar CBCT scans have several specific applications in oral implantology. However, if high-density objects such as titanium dental implants are present within the field of view of the CBCT scan, horizontal image artifacts will be produced.

Beam hardening artifacts are caused due to the differential absorption of low-energy x-ray photons by high-density materials. These artifacts appear as localized hypo-densities or dark voids adjacent to high-density structures, such as titanium implants. The appearance and localization of beam hardening artifacts may be confounded with radiographic aspects of some implant complications. On the other hand, streak artifacts appear as linear hyperdensities radiating from the metallic object that sometimes extend to the entire width of the field.[12-16]

While CBCT effective radiation doses are lower than multi-detector computed tomography,[17-19] they can be significantly higher than 2D intraoral or panoramic radiographs.[17] CBCT techniques and protocols should always be guided by the ALARA and ALADA (as low as diagnostically acceptable)[20] principle. Technical acquisition parameters such as a small field of view (FOV) and small voxel dimensions can be set and optimized to improve image quality. Nevertheless, these protocol changes may also have significant effects on the radiation doses received by the patient.[20-23]

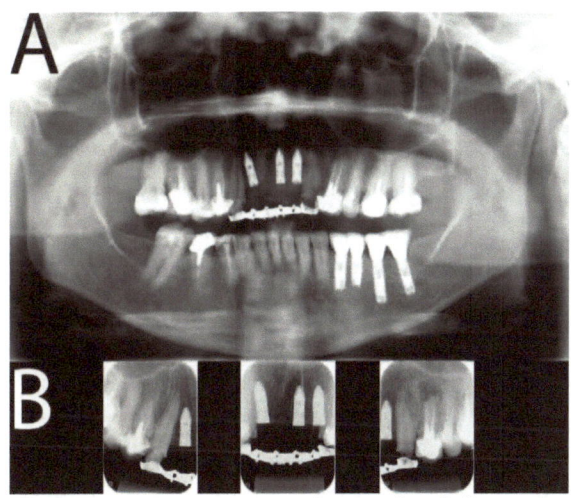

Figure 4-1. *Panoramic radiographic follow-up of multiple implants.*

Follow-up images

According to the most recent guidelines of the American Association of Oral and Maxillofacial Radiologists (AAOMR),[24] digital two-dimensional images (periapical and panoramic radiographs) are still the most recommended for monitoring dental implants of cases that did not present any intrasurgical complications, symptoms related to postoperative infection or radiographic alterations during the follow-up period. The above-mentioned imaging methods are useful to check the bone-implant interface and the stable implant-prosthesis relationship, as well as to follow-up the peri-implant bone level. Panoramic radiographs are indicated to evaluate the overall conditions of multiple implants at the same time, and may be supplemented with periapical radiographs of specific areas, in order to display further details (Figure 4-2).

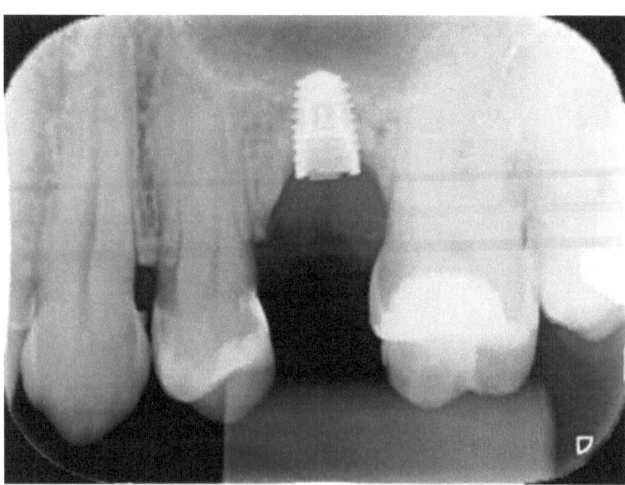

Figure 4-2. *Implant follow-up with periapical radiographs.*

Injuries of anatomic structures

Maxillary sinus floor perforation
Perforation of the maxillary sinus floor (Figure 4-3) occurs generally during drilling of implant sites, or due to maxillary sinus floor augmentation. The main cause of this complication is the inappropriate choice of the radiographic technique used in the diagnosis. Two-dimensional x-ray images present overlapping structures, image magnification and distortion, thus preventing the professional from performing accurate linear measurements. The best

imaging method to assess and follow-up the conditions of the maxillary sinus is the CBCT, which provides full-scale images of sinus anatomical variations such as sinus septa and pneumatization of the maxillary sinus. The main related complications are infections of the maxillary sinuses causing sinusitis, thickening of the sinus mucosa, antral pseudocysts, impaired osseointegration of grafts and implants, and implant displacement into of the maxillary sinus. However, maxillary sinus floor drilling will not always lead to complications.[25]

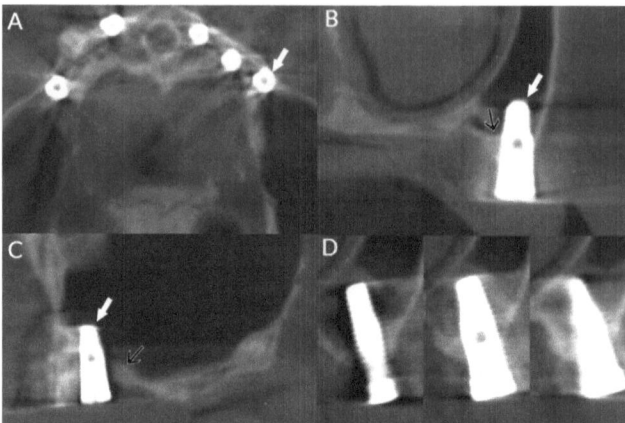

Figure 4-3. *CBCT images showing an implant in the maxillary sinus (arrows). A) Axial view. B) Coronal view. C) Sagittal view. D) Cross-sectional images.*

Nasal cavity perforation
As in the maxillary sinus, perforation of the nasal cavity (Figure 4-4) usually occurs due to the inappropriate choice of the radiographic technique for surgical planning. As explained in the chapter 1, CT and CBCT are the most indicated radiographic examinations for implant planning in all areas of the jaws. Other factors causing this complication are an over-angulation of the implant (Figure 4-5) and severe bone resorption in the region. The most common related postoperative complications are infections, bleeding and impaired osseointegration of implants. On the other hand, some perforations of the floor of the nasal cavity may be asymptomatic.

Injury of nerve canals
Drilling and injury to nerves can occur in both maxilla and mandible. The most common complications in the maxilla involve the nasopalatine canal. Its injury (Figure 4-6) usually occurs due to severe bone

resorption of the alveolar ridge in the anterior region, approaching the area where the implant will be installed and the nasopalatine canal. Anatomical variations (Figure 4-7) not previously detected can also lead to complications.

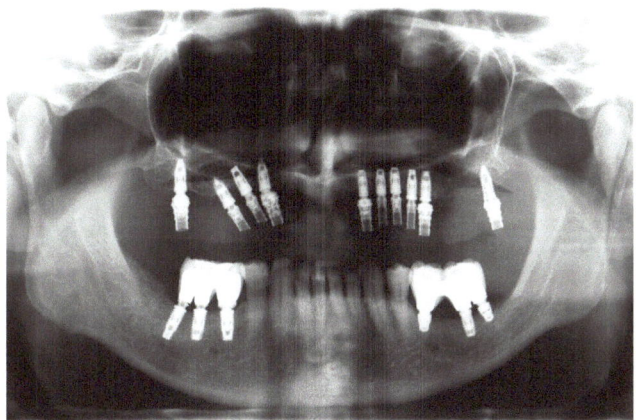

Figure 4-4. *Panoramic radiography showing anterior implants placed in the nasal cavity.*

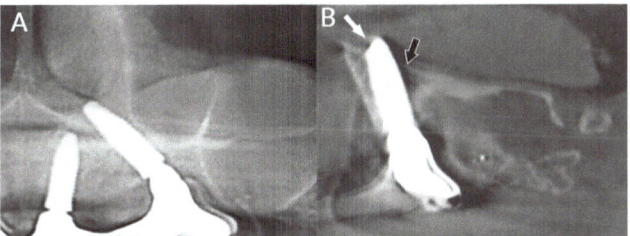

Figure 4-5. *CBCT images showing an implant (white arrow) placed in the nasal cavity. A) Coronal panoramic view. B) Cross-sectional image. Note the nasal floor limit (black arrow).*

The possible consequences of perforating the nasopalatine canal during implant site preparation are not clear, but there are reports of paresthesia after this canal is fenestrated. In the mandible, the mandibular canal and its anatomical variations are the main anatomical structures to be evaluated during the surgical planning, since the mandibular canal injury (Figure 4-8) is not uncommon. It usually occurs due to an inappropriate choice of the radiographic technique for surgical planning, low alveolar bone density, and/or anatomical variations (Figure 4-9) such as accessory and bifid canals. The main consequences are related to the partial or total loss of the injured nerve. The most common are paresthesia and dysesthesia.

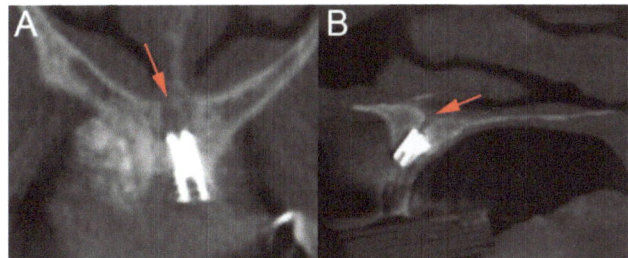

Figure 4-6. *CBCT images showing an implant placed in the nasopalatine canal (red arrow). A) Coronal view. B) Sagittal view.*

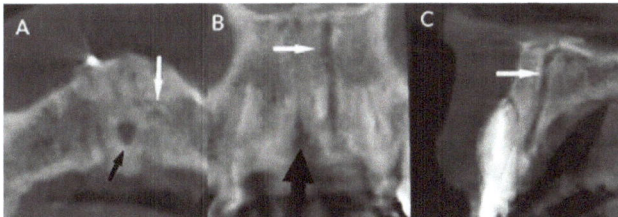

Figure 4-7. *CBCT images showing the anatomical variation named canalis sinuosus (white arrow). A) Axial view. Note the proximity with the nasopalatine canal (black arrow). B) Coronal view. C) Sagittal view.*

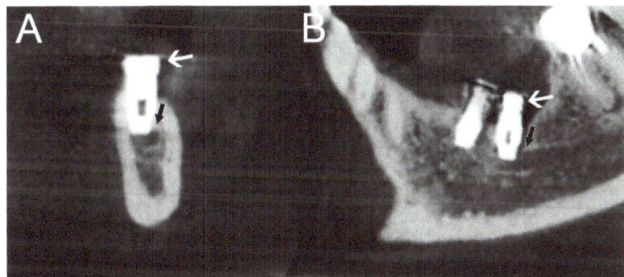

Figure 4-8. *CBCT images showing an implant (white arrow) placed in the mandibular canal (black arrow). A) Cross-sectional image. B) Coronal panoramic view.*

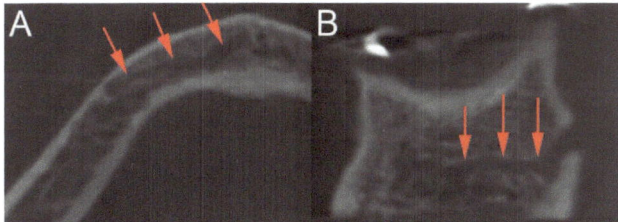

Figure 4-9. *CBCT images showing the mandibular incisive canal (red arrows), which is an anterior extension of the mandibular canal.*

Peri-implant bone loss

Peri-implantitis is one of the most important risk factors in cases of dental implant therapy. In periimplantitis, there is an irreversible inflammation of the peri-implant tissue associated with marginal bone loss (Figure 4-10). This clinical condition differs from peri-implant mucositis cases, in which there is a reversible inflammation of the same tissue, but with no associated bone loss.[3]

Although peri-implantitis has been related to cases with implant loss,[2,4,5] some clinical studies show different results for its frequency. Low rates have recently been found by a clinical study on implant failure after osseointegration. Nevertheless, in another study, a frequency that ranged between 5% and 10% had been found in cases of dental implant rehabilitation.[3]

Jung and collaborators[6] evaluated implant survival rates in cases rehabilitated with implant-supported single crowns. Interestingly, peri-implantitis and soft tissue complications were observed in 9.7% of all cases reviewed. However, only 6.3% of the cases presented marginal bone loss greater than 2mm in the study period.

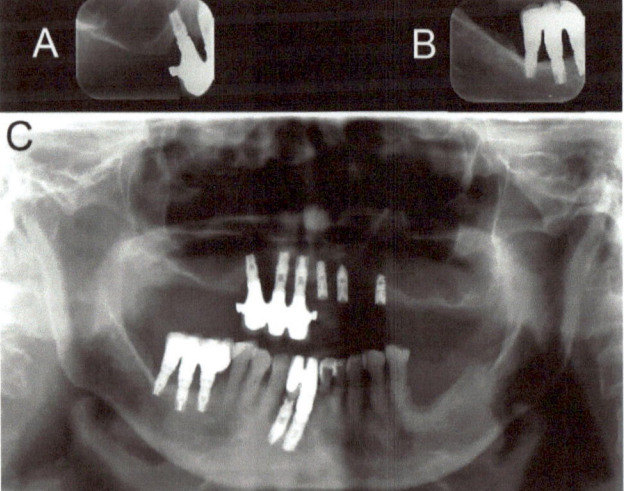

Figure 4-10. Imaging diagnosis of periimplantitis. A) Periapical radiography showing a superior implant with peri-implant bone loss. B) Periapical radiography showing inferior implants with peri-implant bone loss. C) Panoramic radiography of the case.

Detection and follow-up of peri-implant alveolar bone loss are necessary and may influence the course of treatment and its clinical prognosis. While periodontal probing is a very important clinical monitoring procedure, supplemental radiographic imaging should be also considered to assist in establishing a diagnosis. The use of CBCT in the diagnosis of this type of complication (Figure 4-11) is still much discussed. Some studies reported that periapical radiography has a better performance than CBCT.[11,26] On the other hand, more recent studies using CBCT scanners with high resolution acquisition protocols combined with appropriate software tools found a higher reliability of CBCT to diagnose peri-implant bone loss.[16,27,28] Nevertheless the use of CBCT for the diagnosis of peri-implant bone loss is still controversial and must be done carefully, taking into account the effective radiation doses involved.

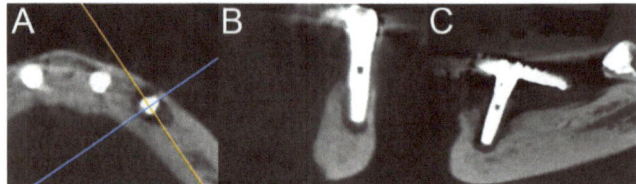

Figure 4-11. CBCT Imaging diagnosis of periimplantitis. A) Axial view. B) Cross-sectional image. C) Coronal Panoramic view.

Alveolar bone fenestration

The fenestration of a bone plate of the alveolar ridge represents an interruption of the cortical plate contour. This is another complication that usually happens by the poor use of images for dental implant planning. In these cases, two-dimensional radiographs may show a false aspect of integrity of the alveolar ridge. Furthermore it is impossible to perform accurate follow-up measurements of the marginal bone level on 2D radiographs.

In the edentulous maxilla, the buccal bone plate usually presents a concave shape due to bone resorption. This is the reason why superior alveolar buccal plates are more susceptible to fenestrations (Figure 4-12). In the mandible, bone resorption pronounces the lingual mandibular bone concavity especially at the submandibular fossa (Figure 4-13). This situation requires precise implant inclinations in order to avoid lingual bone plate fenestration. The consequences of fenestration vary according to the location. The most common are implant mobility, interference with aesthetics, gingival recession and bleeding. In the worst cases, the submandibular gland may also be affected.

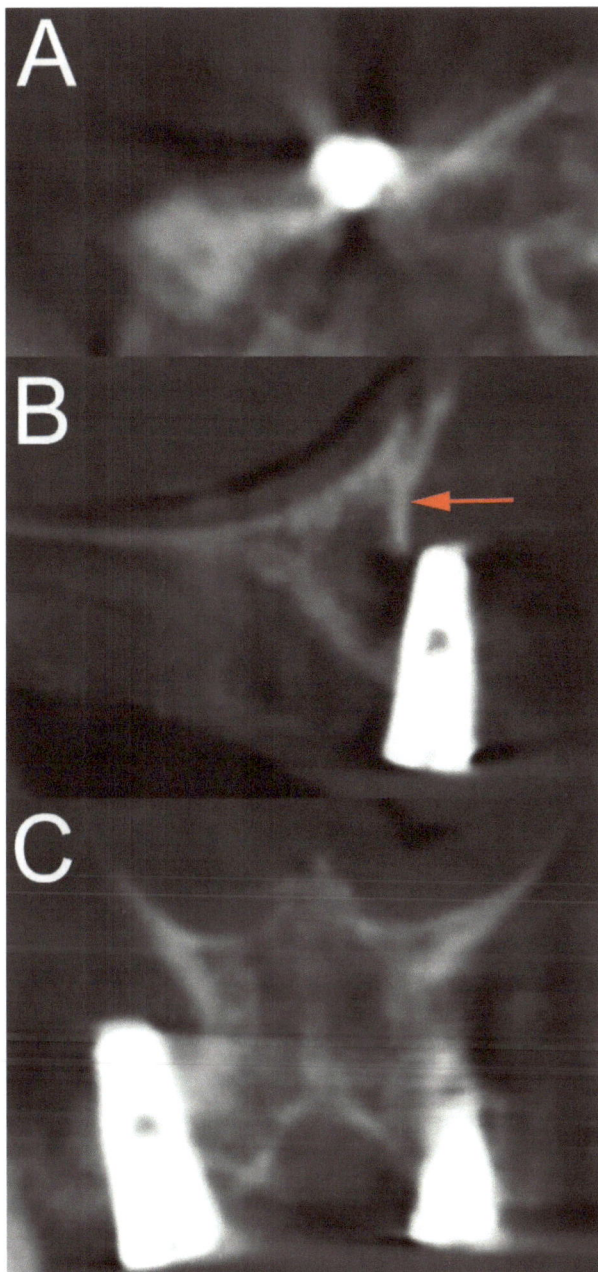

Figure 4-12. *CBCT Imaging diagnosis of a buccal plate (red arrow) fenestration in the maxilla. A) Axial view B) Sagittal view. C) Coronal view.*

Considerations on CBCT parameters

The radiation dose is one of the major concerns related to diagnostic imaging with CT methods. A recent systematic review has reported an update of the term ALARA by the National Commission on Radiation Protection and Measurements. The new term ALADA stands for "as the low diagnostically acceptable". Implementation of this concept will require evidence-based indications to justify the reasons to obtain high-resolution diagnostic images,

taking into consideration the effective radiation doses required to obtain the desired level of quality.[20] This new concept requires the dentist to have a greater knowledge on CBCT acquisition parameters.

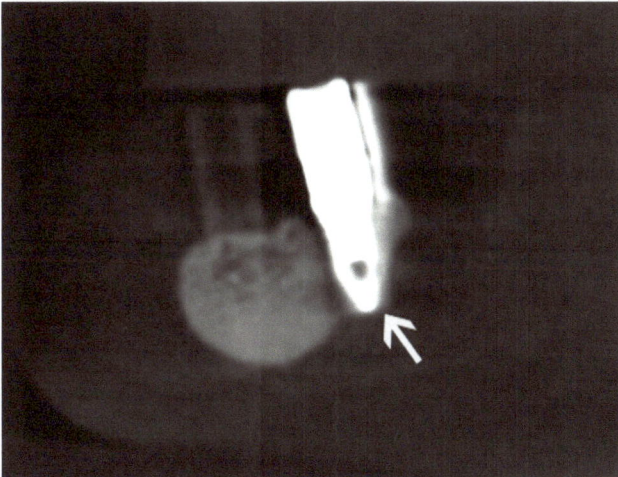

Figure 4-13. *CBCT cross-sectional image of an implant (white arrow) in the submandibular fossa.*

Computed tomographic parameters such as field of view (FOV) size, voxel thickness and number of frames are factors that can directly influence CBCT image quality. A regular diagnostic protocol used for dental implants was described as having a voxel thickness of 0.25 mm, tube voltage of 120kVp, tube current of 8mA, exposure time of 8.5 seconds and field of view of 16 cm in diameter and 6 cm in height.[29] The aforementioned field of view includes only one full dental arch in standard resolution, allowing for a low effective radiation dose (approximately 35 microsieverts), as reported by a study using the i-CAT Classic CBCT device.[30] On the other hand, a recent study using a different device found better detection of peri-implant bone defects using a small FOV (4x4 cm), high number of projection images (1009) and smallest voxel size (0.08 mm nominal resolution).[27]

The radiation doses emitted by CBCT vary among different devices and acquisition protocols. In large FOVs, effective radiation doses may range from 46 to 916 mSv. In average FOVs, doses may range from 47 to 560 mSv. Finally, in small FOVs, doses may range from 39 to 430 mSv.[20] Nevertheless, radiation doses from CBCT are usually less than 10% of the ones from spiral CT scans. Periapical radiography doses, in turn, range from 3 to 5 mSv[17] while panoramic radiography doses may range from 6 to 8 mSv. As a basis of comparison, a round trip flight from Paris to Tokyo exposes the passenger to 150 mSv of cosmic radiation.

Volumetric measurements (segmentation)

The accuracy of CBCT in measuring the volume of osteolytic lesions (i.e. tissue segmentation) was assessed in several studies.[31-34] One of these studies[35] compared the accuracy of CBCT to micro-CT in measuring irregular-shaped cavities created in bovine bone. The authors concluded that CBCT is accurately comparable to micro-CT in assessing artificially created bone cavities, and suggested that it may be a useful tool in conducting endodontic follow-up. Furthermore, Liang and collaborators[31] found a strong correlation between the real volume (obtained by a silicone impression) of artificially created periapical bone defects and their respective CBCT volume measurements.

Therefore, the ability to measure the volume of a lesion intraosseously may provide strong evidences about volume changes and, indirectly, about the healing rate. Furthermore, recent medical articles have evaluated automatic and semi-automatic segmentation methods performed by thresholding algorithms, which could expedite the diagnostic procedure.[35-37]

Manual X Automated tissue segmentation
Manual tissue segmentation is time-consuming and can be influenced by subjective preferences for image interpolation, window levels, and personal bias in regard to where to establish the limits of the lesion, leading to high variability. A recent article described the usefulness of an automated tissue segmentation method based on a region-growing algorithm of a software dedicated for virtual implant planning (ImplantViewer 2.709, Anne Solutions, São Paulo, Brazil).[38] This method is based on gray-scale threshold levels and showed greater reliability in comparison to the manual segmentation. The reason is that fewer corrections and decisions on where to delineate the boundaries of the lesion are necessary. On the other hand, due to connectivity with the periapical lesion, part of the periodontal space is included in the threshold. This may prevent the real volume of a lesion from being calculated accurately.

Nevertheless, greater reliability is still ensured in assessing the lesion's healing rate, since the follow-up evaluations are based on bone changes in the same tooth element.[38]

In the field of oral implantology, segmentation with CBCT has proved useful for volumetric analyses of maxillary sinus grafts.[39] Moreover, despite the fact that both manual and automated segmentations are reliable to calculate the volume of tooth periapical lesions,[38] further clinical studies would still be recommended to address the same role of both methods in cases of implant periapical lesions (Figure 4-14).

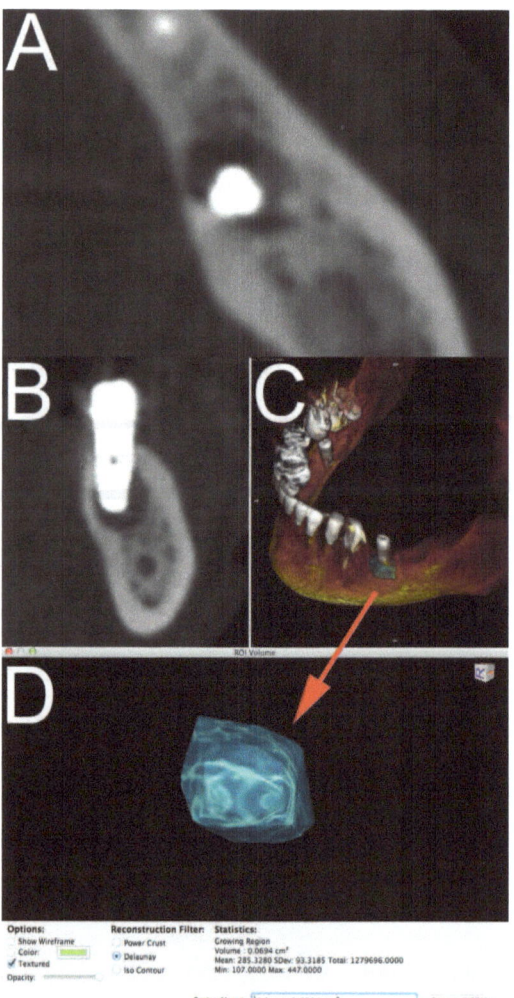

Figure 4-14. *CBCT automated segmentation of an implant periapical lesion using the OsiriX software. A) Axial image showing the buccal-lingual and mesio-distal extensions of the lesion. B) Cross-sectional image showing the buccal-lingual and superior-inferior extensions of the lesion. C) Three-dimensional view of the volume measured. D) Volumetric measurement output.*

Finally, the data reported in this chapter highlight the importance and responsibility of the dental professional in choosing and proper using the most adequate radiographic examination for planning implant surgeries. The majority of the complications involving dental implants have origin in the surgical planning phase. Therefore, the dentist should always have technical and scientific knowledge to proper use radiographic methods while also protecting the patient against excessive radiation doses.

Follow-up of grafting procedures

The importance of the clinical and radiographic diagnosis and postoperative evaluation of grafting surgeries has already been described in the literature.[41] If used according to the ALARA guidelines, CBCT can be an appropriate image-obtaining method, indicated for 3D assessments of treatments related to implant placement and reconstructive dentistry (Figures 4-15 and 4-16), since planned grafted and implant sites have to be reconstructed in terms of both height and width.[40]

Nevertheless, because dental implantology is inherently dealing with metallic bodies, related CBCT cuts may show beam-hardening artifacts, which are caused by backprojecting an intensity measured but not corresponding to the actual absorption because mainly high-energetic X-rays penetrate the relatively dense implant.[41] CBCT follow-up axial images (Figure 4-17) of reconstructive treatments with grafts and multiple implants usually shows beam-hardening artifacts between implants.[42]

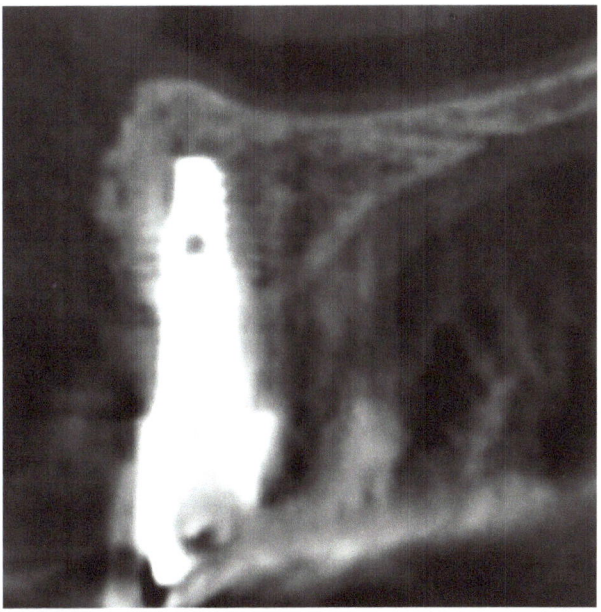

Figure 4-15. *CBCT cross-sectional image of an implant placed in an area grafted with onlay blocks, after a 7-year follow-up.*

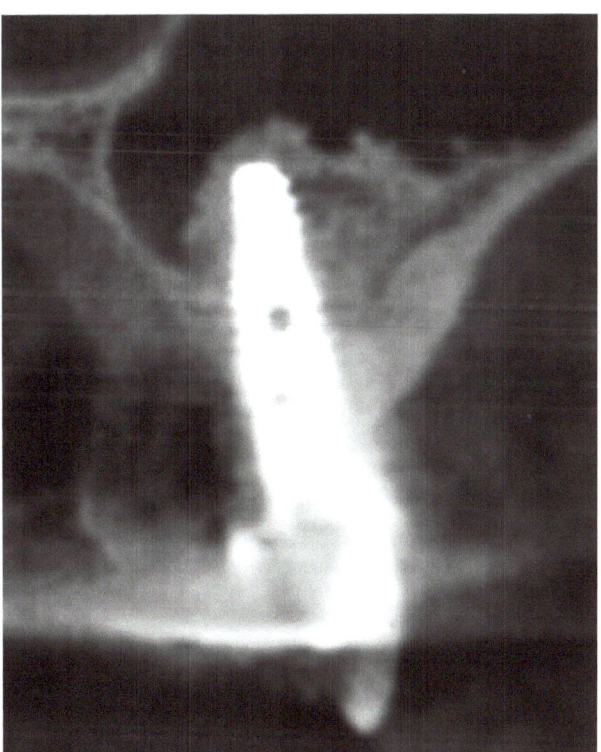

Figure 4-16. *CBCT cross-sectional image of an implant placed in a sinus grafted area, after a 7-year follow-up.*

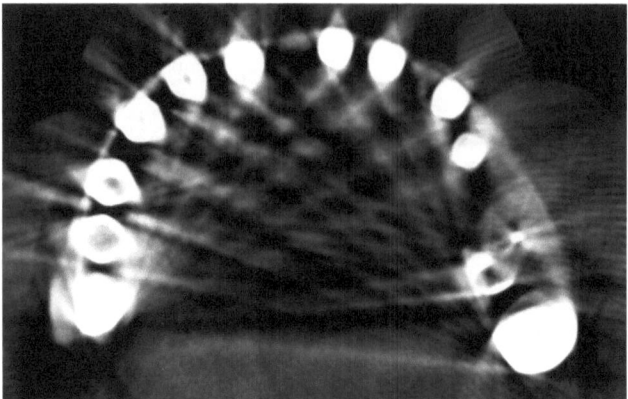

Figure 4-17. *CBCT axial image of maxillary implants placed in grafted areas. Note the beam-hardening artifacts between implants.*

References

1. Albrektsson T, Jansson T, Lekholm U. Osseointegrated dental implants. Dent Clin North Am. 1986;30(1):151-74.

2. Busenlechner D, Furhauser R, Haas R, Watzek G, Mailath G, Pommer B. Long-term implant success at the Academy for Oral Implantology: 8-year follow-up and risk factor analysis. J Periodontal Implant Sci. 2014;44(3):102-8.

3. Daubert DM, Weinstein BF, Bordin S, Leroux BG, Flemming TF. Prevalence and predictive factors for peri-implant disease and implant failure: a cross-sectional analysis. Journal of periodontology. 2015;86(3):337-47.

4. Romanos GE, Javed F, Delgado-Ruiz RA, Calvo-Guirado JL. Peri-implant diseases: a review of treatment interventions. Dent Clin North Am. 2015;59(1):157-78.

5. Padial-Molina M, Suarez F, Rios HF, Galindo-Moreno P, Wang HL. Guidelines for the diagnosis and treatment of peri-implant diseases. Int J Periodontics Restorative Dent. 2014;34(6):e102-11.

6. De Smet E, Jacobs R, Gijbels F, Naert I. The accuracy and reliability of radiographic methods for the assessment of marginal bone level around oral implants. Dento maxillo facial radiology. 2002;31(3):176-81.

7. Schliephake H, Wichmann M, Donnerstag F, Vogt S. Imaging of periimplant bone levels of implants with buccal bone defects. Clin Oral Implants Res. 2003;14(2):193-200.

8. Kavadella A, Karayiannis A, Nicopoulou-Karayianni K. Detectability of experimental peri-implant cancellous bone lesions using conventional and direct digital radiography. Aust Dent J. 2006;51(2):180-6.

9. Mengel R, Kruse B, Flores-de-Jacoby L. Digital volume tomography in the diagnosis of peri-implant defects: an in vitro study on native pig mandibles. Journal of periodontology. 2006;77(7):1234-41.

10. Kullman L, Al-Asfour A, Zetterqvist L, Andersson L. Comparison of radiographic bone height assessments in panoramic and intraoral radiographs of implant patients. The International journal of oral & maxillofacial implants. 2007;22(1):96-100.

11. Sirin Y, Horasan S, Yaman D, Basegmez C, Tanyel C, Aral A, et al. Detection of crestal radiolucencies around dental implants: an in vitro experimental study. J Oral Maxillofac Surg. 2012;70(7):1540-50.

12. Barrett JF, Keat N. Artifacts in CT: recognition and avoidance. Radiographics. 2004;24(6):1679-91.

13. Schulze RK, Berndt D, d'Hoedt B. On cone-beam computed tomography artifacts induced by titanium implants. Clin Oral Implants Res. 2010;21(1):100-7.

14. Schulze R, Heil U, Gross D, Bruellmann DD, Dranischnikow E, Schwanecke U, et al. Artefacts in CBCT: a review. Dento maxillo facial radiology. 2011;40(5):265-73.

15. Angelopoulos C, Scarfe WC, Farman AG. A comparison of maxillofacial CBCT and medical CT. Atlas of the oral and maxillofacial surgery clinics of North America. 2012;20(1):1-17.

16. Kamburoglu K, Murat S, Kilic C, Yuksel S, Avsever H, Farman A, et al. Accuracy of CBCT images in the assessment of buccal marginal alveolar peri-implant defects: effect of field of view. Dento maxillo facial radiology. 2014;43(4):20130332.

17. Patel S. New dimensions in endodontic imaging: Part 2. Cone beam computed tomography. Int Endod J. 2009;42(6):463-75.

18. Costa FF, Gaia BF, Umetsubo OS, Cavalcanti MG. Detection of horizontal root fracture with small-volume cone-beam computed tomography in the presence and absence of intracanal metallic post. J Endod. 2011;37(10):1456-9.

19. Cavalcanti MG. Cone beam computed tomographic imaging: perspective, challenges, and the impact of near-trend future applications. J Craniofac Surg. 2012;23(1):279-82.

20. Ludlow JB, Timothy R, Walker C, Hunter R, Benavides E, Samuelson DB, et al. Effective dose of dental CBCT-a meta analysis of published data and

additional data for nine CBCT units. Dento maxillo facial radiology. 2015;44(1):20140197.

21. Costa FF, Gaia BF, Umetsubo OS, Pinheiro LR, Tortamano IP, Cavalcanti MG. Use of large-volume cone-beam computed tomography in identification and localization of horizontal root fracture in the presence and absence of intracanal metallic post. J Endod. 2012;38(6):856-9.

22. de-Azevedo-Vaz SL, Vasconcelos Kde F, Neves FS, Melo SL, Campos PS, Haiter-Neto F. Detection of periimplant fenestration and dehiscence with the use of two scan modes and the smallest voxel sizes of a cone-beam computed tomography device. Oral Surg Oral Med Oral Pathol Oral Radiol. 2013;115(1):121-7.

23. Bornstein MM, Scarfe WC, Vaughn VM, Jacobs R. Cone beam computed tomography in implant dentistry: a systematic review focusing on guidelines, indications, and radiation dose risks. The International journal of oral & maxillofacial implants. 2014;29 Suppl:55-77.

24. Tyndall DA, Price JB, Tetradis S, Ganz SD, Hildebolt C, Scarfe WC, et al. Position statement of the American Academy of Oral and Maxillofacial Radiology on selection criteria for the use of radiology in dental implantology with emphasis on cone beam computed tomography. Oral Surg Oral Med Oral Pathol Oral Radiol. 2012;113(6):817-26.

25. Tamimi DF. Specialty Imaging: Dental Implants: AMIRSYS; 2014. 472 p.

26. Dave M, Davies J, Wilson R, Palmer R. A comparison of cone beam computed tomography and conventional periapical radiography at detecting peri-implant bone defects. Clin Oral Implants Res. 2013;24(6):671-8.

27. Pinheiro LR, Scarfe WC, de Oliveira Sales MA, Gaia BF, Cortes AR, Cavalcanti MG. Effect of Cone Beam Computed Tomography Field of View and Acquisition Frames on the Detection of Chemically Simulated Peri-Implant Bone Loss in Vitro. Journal of periodontology. 2015:1-11.

28. Ritter L, Elger MC, Rothamel D, Fienitz T, Zinser M, Schwarz F, et al. Accuracy of peri-implant bone evaluation using cone beam CT, digital intra-oral radiographs and histology. Dento maxillo facial radiology. 2014;43(6):20130088.

29. Cortes AR, Eimar H, Barbosa J de S, Costa C, Arita ES, Tamimi F. Sensitivity and specificity of radiographic methods for predicting insertion torque of dental implants. J Periodontol. 2015;86(5):646-55.

30. Roberts JA, Drage NA, Davies J, Thomas DW. Effective dose from cone beam CT examinations in dentistry. Br J Radiol 2009;82:35-40.

31. Liang YH, Jiang L, Gao XJ, Shemesh H, Wesselink PR, Wu MK. Detection and measurement of artificial periapical lesions by cone-beam computed tomography. Int Endod J. 2014;47:332-338.

32. Ahlowalia MS, Patel S, Anwar HM, Cama G, Austin RS, Wilson R, et al. Accuracy of CBCT for volumetric measurement of simulated periapical lesions. Int Endod J. 2013;46:538-546.

33. Pinsky HM, Dyda S, Pinsky RW, Misch KA, Sarment DP. Accuracy of three-dimensional measurements using cone-beam CT. Dentomaxillofac Radiol. 2006;35:410-416.

34. Wang Y, He S, Guo Y, Wang S, Chen S. Accuracy of volumetric measurement of simulated root resorption lacunas based on cone beam computed tomography. Orthod Craniofac Res. 2013;16:169-176.

35. Rosenbluth KH, Gimenez F, Kells AP, Salegio EA, Mittermeyer GM, Modera K, et al. Automated segmentation tool for brain infusions. PloS One. 2013;8:e64452.

36. Thierfelder KM, Sommer WH, Baumann AB, Klotz E, Meinel FG, Strobl FF, et al. Whole-brain CT perfusion: reliability and reproducibility of volumetric perfusion deficit assessment in patients with acute ischemic stroke. Neuroradiol. 2013;55:827-835.

37. Yang X, Yu HC, Choi Y, Lee W, Wang B, Yang J, et al. A hybrid semi-automatic method for liver segmentation based on level-set methods using multiple seed points. Comput Methods Programs Biomed. 2014;113:69-79.

38. Aoki EM, Abdala-Júnior R, Oliveira JX, Arita ES, Cortes AR. Reliability and Reproducibility of Manual and Automated Volumetric Measurements of Periapical Lesions. J Endod 2015;30:pii: S0099-2399(15)00578-6.

39. Kim ES, Moon SY, Kim SG, Park HC, Oh JS. Three-dimensional volumetric analysis after sinus grafts. Implant Dent 2013;22(2):170-4.

40. Acocella A, Sacco R, Niardi P, et al. Early implant placement in bilateral sinus floor augmentation using iliac bone block grafts in severe maxillary

atrophy: a clinical, histological, and radiographic case report. J Oral Implantol 2009;35:37-44.

41. Schulze RK, Berndt D, d'Hoedt B. On cone-beam computed tomography artifacts induced by titanium implants. Clin Oral Implants Res 2010;21:100-107.

CHAPTER 5

LATERAL RIDGE AUGMENTATION: PARTICULATE BONE GRAFTS

Arthur Rodriguez Gonzalez Cortes

Loss of ridge width due to bone resorption is a common event in patients with tooth loss, and may be presented with varying degrees.[1] After tooth extraction, socket remodeling may result in loss of up to 60% of the alveolar ridge width within the first two years.[2] Complications may worsen if there is damage to the buccal plate during tooth removal. In these cases, even if an implant-supported crown can be installed, irregular bony anatomy may lead to an unnatural appearance of the final crown.

There are some ways to solve such problems with minimal trauma, such as lateral alveolar ridge augmentation with particulate graft, and use of bone expanders. The development of surgical techniques has increased the number of ways to achieve a successful result.[3,4] Nevertheless, pre-existing bone resorption still remains an important challenge in sites where implant placement is required. Although ridge augmentation with block grafts can help restore ridge volume, harvesting autogenous bone can significantly increase treatment time and costs and also pose risks such as nerve or arterial injury, postoperative pain and infection.[5-9]

One of the solutions to place dental implants in cases of severe alveolar atrophy is the ridge-splitting technique, which allows the ridge to be widened by a less invasive procedure than the traditional bone block grafting approaches. However, ridge splitting requires a complicated surgery that involves a purposeful longitudinal fracture made to split the crest in the middle.[10-12]

The use of osteotomes of increasing diameter has also been described as a method to place implants in the maxilla with poor bone density, although it is difficult to be performed in the posterior maxilla due to limited mouth opening. Furthermore, the osteotome technique also requires the exertion of some force for which the amount and direction are not fully controllable.[13-15]

Another option described in the literature is the technique of lateral bone expansion using screws of increasing diameter. This is a technique that aims at achieving bone expansion with minimal levels of trauma.[16,17]

Guided Bone Regeneration (GBR)

Guided bone regeneration is considered a safe surgical procedure commonly used to perform lateral ridge augmentation. This technique can be performed right after tooth extraction to prevent bone loss, on healed alveolar ridges before implant placement to augment ridge width, or even during implant placement surgeries, in cases of buccal dehiscences or ridge contour defects. CT or CBCT cross-sectional images are required to determine the need for GBR. Cases with lack of alveolar bone width only at the alveolar crest will have better prognosis than cases with horizontal deficiencies at both crestal and apical levels. Success in achieving new bone formation using this procedure in cases of ridge width augmentation associated with dental implant placement has been attributed to the using of barrier membranes to create a secluded anatomic site (Figure 5-1). This technique has been extensively documented by clinical and histological studies in the literature.[18-20]

In the GBR procedure, particulate grafts are always followed by the placement of a resorbable collagen membrane to mechanically prevent the undesirable penetration of fibroblasts and epithelial cells to the bone defect area, creating a secluded space where bone regeneration may occur. When necessary, release of the periosteum can also be performed to obtain a tension-free closure. With this procedure, osteogenic cell populations from the parent bone are prompted to stimulate new bone formation in the bone defect area by the mechanical exclusion of undesirable soft tissue, thus preventing it from growing into the osseous defect.[21,22]

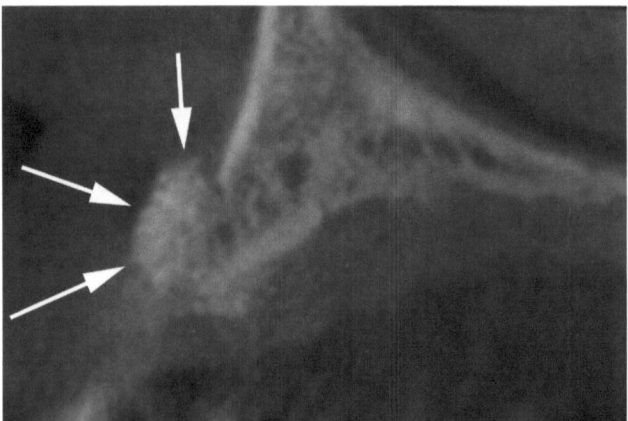

Figure 5-1. CBCT cross-sectional image showing the aspect of a GBR case after healing of the particulate graft (Straumann BoneCeramic®, Institut Straumann AG, Basel, Switzerland). Note the limits of the augmented buccal plate (white arrows).

Esthetic Grafting

Despite the development of GBR, a number of techniques for grafting buccal plates without barrier membranes for lateral augmentation have also been described in the literature.[23-27] One of these surgical techniques is named Esthetic Grafting. It is indicated to correct buccal bone defects, in order to improve hard and soft tissue contours during dental implant placement surgeries (Figure 5-2). A clinical study observed treatment success in cases of sites with satisfactory soft tissue volume, within a 2-year follow-up.[23] Furthermore, a soft tissue thickness of at least 2 mm has been indicated as an important clinical prerequisite to avoid peri-implant bone loss.[28]

In the Esthetic Grafting technique, a crestal incision is performed slightly palatal to the crest midline, followed by elevation of the mucogingival flap, surgical preparation of the implant site, proper implant placement and positioning of the healing screw. Then, the buccal bone defect that remains after performing the dental implant placement can be immediately and completely grafted with a particulate graft material to avoid exposure of the implant body, and to obtain a natural buccal ridge contour. The dental implant site should then be overcorrected buccally with the same graft material, whereby the buccal-lingual width can be expanded at the implant site by at least 2 mm. In contrast with the GBR technique, the bone site receiving esthetic grafting is covered only by the sutured flap tissue.[23] If necessary, the periosteum can be released to obtain a tension-free closure. After the implant healing period, implants are restored and followed up. This technique has been described as useful in cases of delayed and immediate dental implant placement.[29]

In this type of surgery, it is suggested that a potential barrier function is performed by the periosteum.[27] However, a larger amount of graft material is required in order to slightly overcorrect the buccal defect, since resorption and apical migration of the graft material are expected.[23] On the other hand, buccal dehiscences presented around immediate implants are usually presented as three-wall defects, whose prognoses are considered better than that of one-wall defects, frequently observed in cases of severely resorbed ridge.

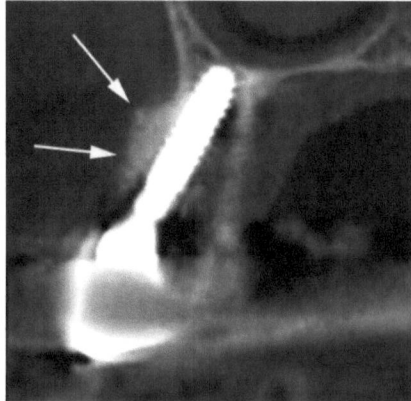

Figure 5-2. CBCT cross-sectional image of a case treated with Esthetic Grafting, performed with a biphasic calcium phosphate material (Straumann BoneCeramic®) to correct ridge contour immediately after implant placement. Note the aspect of the grafted buccal plate (white arrows) after healing of the particulate graft.

Ridge-splitting technique

Ridge-splitting is a surgical technique that creates a space in the alveolar ridge by splitting the alveolar crest in two parts. CBCT images are useful to make longitudinal and horizontal measurements, in order to help the surgeon to define the line where the ridge should be split. Ridge-splitting can also be performed simultaneously with implant placement. Particulate graft materials can then be used to fill the voids around the implants in the widened alveolar crest. Although it involves a more traumatic and complicated surgery, this technique is useful in atrophic edentulous maxillae (Figure 5-3), providing ridge widening through the entire ridge area.[12] It also reduces procedure times as well as the number of surgical procedures required. Furthermore, the procedure can also be performed with piezoelectric surgery, with minimal trauma and faster procedure times.

The surgical technique of ridge-splitting requires a one-centimeter penetration of an osteotome blade in the alveolar ridge crest, which may cause some lateral ridge expansion by itself. The position and depth reached by the osteotome blade can also be measured on CBCT images using the linear measurement tool.

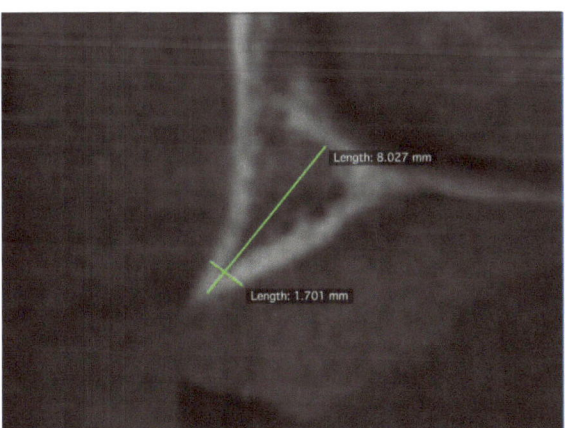

Figure 5-3. CBCT cross-sectional image of an atrophic maxilla representing an indication for the ridge-splitting technique.

Lateral bone expansion with screws

This is a technique that requires a nontraumatic bone expansion kit, which is basically composed of a few screw-assisted bone expanders (Figure 5-4) of increasing diameter, a carrier, and a ratchet. This type of screws has a conical shape so that the diameter increases as maximum depth is reached. The screws must always be used carefully, after the use of the first cylindrical drill for the preparation of the implant site, which follows the desired depth of the osteotomy, according to the length of the implant to be used.

This technique has been described to allow the professional to expand the ridge up to 5 mm of crestal thickness. Results could be previewed in CT images using area and linear measurement tools of the CT software. In cases with fenestration of the remaining bone, particulate grafts could also be used to correct bone contour defects.

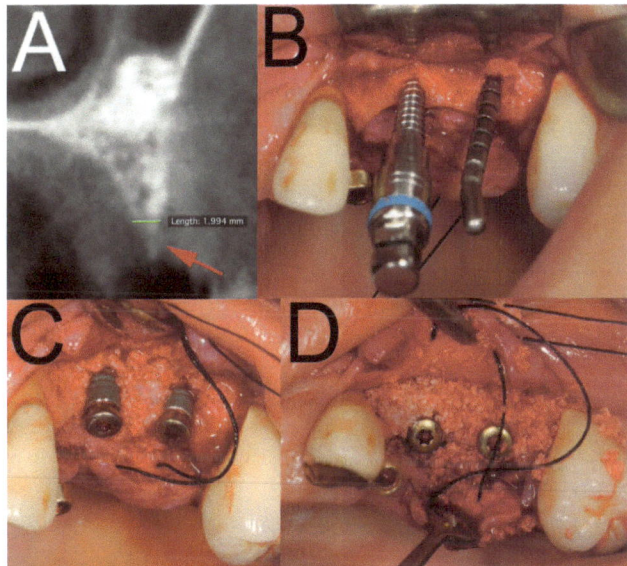

Figure 5-4. Screw-assisted bone expansion. A) CBCT cross-sectional imaging of an implant site that had undergone sinus floor augmentation. Note the lack of buccal-lingual bone thickness at the crest level (red arrow). B) Screw-assisted bone expander positioned at the left maxillary first premolar site. C) Two Straumann Bone Level implants (3.3 x 12 mm) were placed. Note the buccal dehiscence defects. D) The buccal dehiscence defects were corrected with particulate grafts.

50

References

1. Atwood DA, Coy WA. Clinical, cephalometric, and densitometric study of reduction in residual ridges. J Prosthet Dent 1971;26:280-295.

2. Johnson K. A study of the dimensional changes occurring in the maxilla following tooth extraction.1. Branemark PI. Osseointegration and its experimental background. J Prosthet Dent 1983;50:399-410.

3. Romeo E, Chiapasco M, Ghisolfi M, Vogel G. Long term clinical effectiveness of oral implants in the treatment of partial edentulism: Seven year life table analysis of a prospective study with ITI dental implants system used for single tooth restoration. Clin Oral Implants Res 2002;13:133-43.

4. Garg AK, Morales MJ, Navarro I, et al. Autogenous mandibular bone grafts in the treatment of the resorbed maxillary anterior alveolar ridge: Rationale and approach. Implant Dent 1998;7:169-76.

5. Cranin AN, Katzap M, Demirdjan E, et al. Autogenous bone ridge augmentation using the mandibular symphysis as a donor. J Oral Implantol 2001;27:43-7.

6. Li J, Wang HL. Common implant-related advanced bone grafting complications: classification, etiology, and management. Implant Dent 2008;17:389-401.

7. Sjöström M, Sennerby L, Nilson H, et al. Reconstruction of the atrophic edentulous maxilla with free iliac crest grafts and implants: A 3-year report of a prospective clinical study. Clin Implant Dent Relat Res 2007;9:46-59.

8. Stellingsma C, Vissink A, Meijer HJ, et al. Implantology and the severely resorbed edentulous mandible. Crit Rev Oral Biol Med 2004;15:240-8.

9. Shimoyama T, Kaneko T, Shimizu S, et al. Ridge widening and immediate implant placement: A case report. Implant Dent 2001;10:108-112.

11. Simion M, Saldoni M, Zaffe D. Jawbone enlargement using immediate implant placement associated with a split crest technique and guided tissue regeneration. Int J Periodontics Restorative Dent 1992;2:462-73.

12. Guirado JL, Yuguero MR, Carrio´ n del Valle MJ, et al. A maxillary ridgesplitting technique followed by immediate placement of implants: A case report. Implant Dent 2005;14:14-20.

13. Summers RB. A new concept in maxillary implant surgery: The osteotome technique. Compendium 1994;15:152-60.

14. Demarosi F, Leghissa GC, Sardella A, et al. Localised maxillary ridge expansion with simultaneous implant placement: a case series. Br J Oral Maxillofac Surg 2009;47:535-40.

15. Santagata M, Guariniello L, D'Andrea A, et al. Single-tooth replacement in the esthetic zone with ridge expansion osteotomy: A clinical report and radiographic results. J Oral Implantol 2008;34:219-22.

16. Siddiqui AA, Sosovicka M. Lateral bone condensing and expansion for placement of endosseous dental implants: A new technique. J Oral Implantol 2006;32:87-94.

17. Cortes, AR, Cortes DN. Nontraumatic Bone Expansion for Immediate Dental Implant Placement: An Analysis of 21 Cases. Implant Dent 2010;19:92-7.

18. Simion M, Scarano A, Gionso L, Piattelli A. Guided bone regeneration using resorbable and nonresorbable membranes: a comparative histologic study in humans. Int J Oral Maxillofac Implants 1996;11:735-42.

19. Mayfield L, Nobréus N, Attström R, Linde A. Guided bone regeneration in dental implant treatment using a bioabsorbable membrane. Clin Oral Implants Res 1997;8:10-7.

20. Lorenzoni M, Pertl C, Polansky RA, Jakse N, Wegscheider WA. Evaluation of implants placed with barrier membranes. A retrospective follow-up study up to five years. Clin Oral Implants Res 2002;13:274-80.

21. Dahlin C, Linde A, Gottlow J, Nyman S. Healing of bone defects by guided tissue regeneration. Plast Reconstr Surg 1988;81:672-6.

22. Hjørting-Hansen E, Helbo M, Aaboe M, Gotfredsen K, Pinholt EM. Osseointegration of subperiosteal implant via guided tissue regeneration. A pilot study. Clin Oral Implants Res 1995;6:149-54.

23. Le B, Burstein J. Esthetic grafting for small volume hard and soft tissue contour defects for implant site development. Implant Dent 2008;17:136-141.

24. Block MS, Degen M. Horizontal ridge augmentation using human mineralized particulate bone: Preliminary results. J Oral Maxillofac Surg 2004;62(9 suppl 2):67-72.

25. Block MS. Horizontal ridge augmentation using particulate bone. Atlas Oral Maxillofac Surg Clin North Am 2006;14:27-38.

26. Le B, Burstein J, Sedghizadeh PP. Cortical tenting grafting technique in the severely atrophic alveolar ridge for implant site preparation. Implant Dent 2008;17:40-50.

27. Park SH, Lee KW, Oh TJ, Misch CE, Shotwell J, Wang HL. Effect of absorbable membranes on sandwich bone augmentation. Clin Oral Implants Res 2008;19:32-41.

28. Linkevicius T, Apse P, Grybauskas S, Puisys A. The influence of soft tissue thickness on crestal bone changes around implants: a 1-year prospective controlled clinical trial. Int J Oral Maxillofac Implants 2009;24:712-9.

29. Cortes AR, Cortes DN, Arita ES. Correction of buccal dehiscence at the time of implant placement without using barrier membranes: A retrospective cone beam computed tomographic study. Int J Oral Maxillofac Implants. 2013;28:1564-69.

CHAPTER 6

BLOCK BONE GRAFTS

Jesus Torres García-Denche
Faleh Tamimi
Arthur Rodriguez Gonzalez Cortes

Bone regeneration procedures in implant dentistry

In daily dental clinical practice, it is common to find situations in which the bone volume is insufficient for an ideal dental implant placement. Alveolar bone augmentation provides the solution necessary in these cases. Procedures such as sinus lifting and alveolar ridge augmentation have reached high levels of predictability, becoming important in implant dentistry. Bone autograft, alone or in combination with other bone substitutes, has been the biomaterial of choice for clinicians worldwide due its good osteoconductive and osteoinductive properties.[1-3] However, several different xenogeneic, allogeneic and synthetic biomaterials have shown promising results in alveolar bone augmentation procedures.[4-6]

The increasing interest of clinicians and researchers in bone augmentation procedures and biomaterials stems from the fact that about 10-20% of the patients that need treatments with dental implants also require additional bone regeneration procedures before dental implant placement. Bone regeneration procedures are becoming common in the daily practice of dentistry around the world as a result of the wide acceptance of dental implants as one of the main options for oral rehabilitation. Bone regeneration procedures are critical for the success of dental implant treatments in cases where there is a deficiency in bone width and/or height.

The term "bone graft" was defined as: "any implanted material that alone or in combination with other materials promotes a bone healing response by providing osteogenic, osteoinductive or osteoconductive properties".[7] Also, an osteogenic material can be defined as a material that has inherent capacity to form bone, which implies to contain living cells that can be differentiated into bone cells. An osteoinductive material provides biologic signals capable to induce local cells to enter a pathway of differentiation leading to mature osteoblasts. An osteoconductive biomaterial, in turn, provides a three-dimensional and interconnected scaffold where local bone tissue may regenerate new living bone. However, osteoconductive biomaterials are unable to directly induce new bone formation.

Another property of the most used bone graft substitutes is the biodegradability. This is defined as the capacity of degradation of a particle by two main mechanisms: passive chemical degradation or dissolution; and active cellular activity mediated by osteoclast and/or macrophages. Moreover, the biological properties of bone substitute biomaterials are influenced by their porosity, surface geometry and surface chemistry. The events leading to bone healing and regeneration are also influenced by all the variables mentioned above. However, host factors such as bone quality and vascularity of the graft recipient site may also influence the final outcome of a bone regeneration procedure with a bone substitute.

The bone graft material needed for each bone regeneration procedure must be selected based on the material characteristics, and on the surgical procedure itself. Some factors such as osteogenic potential of the host residual bone, systemic health of patients, and morphology of the bone defects should be considered in the choice of bone substitute for each situation.

Onlay bone grafts

Autogenous bone graft

Bone augmentation using autogenous onlay bone grafts, harvested from either intraoral or extraoral sources is considered to be a reliable technique with high success rates and satisfactory histological results.[8,9] The cellular component of trabecular bone graft includes few osteoblasts and a high number of precursor cells that survive the transplantation. These precursor cells, in turn, are responsible for the osteogenic potential of bone autograft. In this context, intraoral grafts are always preferred, since they tend to resorb less than extraoral bone grafts after implantation.[10] However, autogenous onlay grafts have some disadvantages, which might limit patient's acceptance to the treatment, including unpredictable bone resorption rates and limited availability, as well as postoperative pain and bleeding associated with the harvesting surgery.[11,12] On the other hand, long-term satisfactory results with this technique are achievable, provided that proper clinical follow-up and maintenance are performed. Accordingly, implant survival rates higher than 90% have been described by literature reviews on onlay grafts.[13]

The main indication of onlay bone grafts is to overcome extreme loss of ridge bone thickness (Figures 6-1 to 6-4). Gains of approximately 5 mm in alveolar bone width and height have been reported by studies using autogenous onlay grafts with satisfactory implant survival rates.[9,13,14] Grafts have the potential to induce osteoconduction, as well as to enable healing in the recipient site.[10]

In cases where it is not possible to use autografts, onlay bone grafting could be performed using biomaterials with block shapes, which are directly placed onto the host bone surface and covered with the flap tissue. This procedure requires a biomaterial strong enough to bear direct occlusal forces and to be fixed in the bone with a screw. Besides, biomaterials should also be bioresorbable and osteoconductive. Several animals studies have

shown that blocks made of either allogeneic bone graft materials, hydroxyapatite, triphasic calcium phosphates or monetite are capable of achieving vertical bone augmentation in onlay bone graft procedures.[15-17] Another alternative to autografts for onlay bone grafting is the use of allogeneic bone blocks, which have also proved useful in clinical studies.[18]

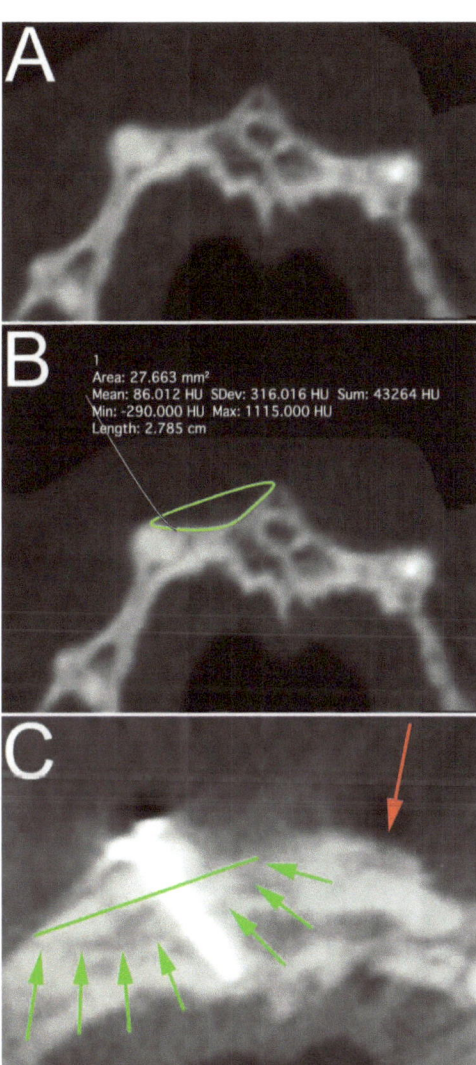

Figure 6-1. *Autogenous onlay block graft in the right anterior maxilla. A) Initial CBCT axial image. Two block grafts were planned to restore the anterior maxilla. B) Volumetric surgical planning of the right block graft. C) CBCT axial image of the block grafts obtained after a 6-month healing period. Note the estimation of the initial surgical plan (green line) and the limit between right block graft and host bone (green arrows). The left block graft (red arrow) had also been installed in the same surgery.*

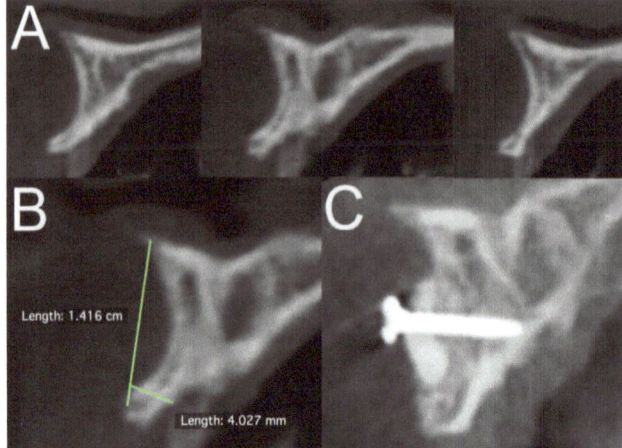

Figure 6-2. *CBCT cross-sectional images of the case depicted in Figure 6-1. A) Initial cross-sectional images of the right anterior maxilla. B) Volumetric surgical plan estimating an ideal final aspect of the site. C) Cross-sectional image of the right block graft obtained after a six-month healing period.*

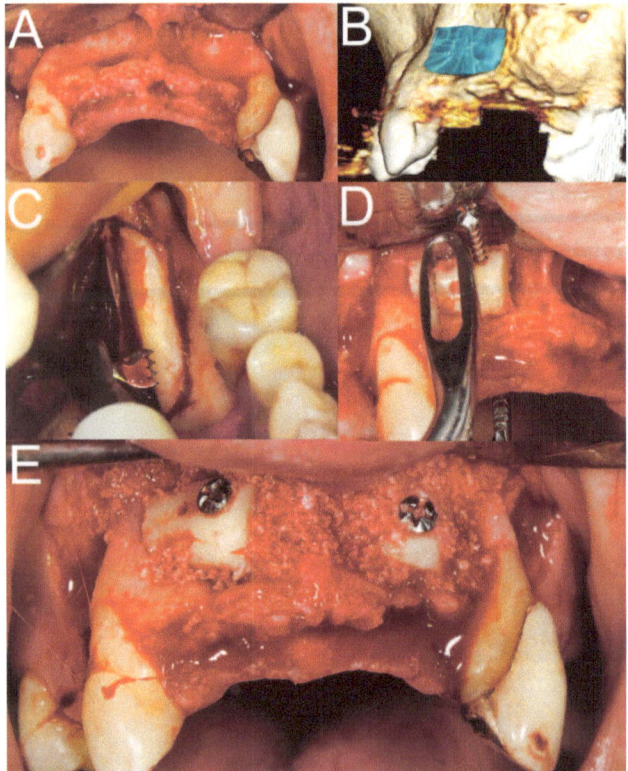

Figure 6-3. *Clinical aspects of the block graft installation depicted in Figures 6-1 and 6-2. A) Initial clinical view of the anterior maxilla. B) Volumetric estimation of the amount of bone graft required. C) Bone harvesting from the mandibular ramus. D) Right block graft installation. E) Particulate synthetic graft (Straumann BoneCeramic®, Institut Straumann AG, Basel, Switzerland) was used in association with the block grafts.*

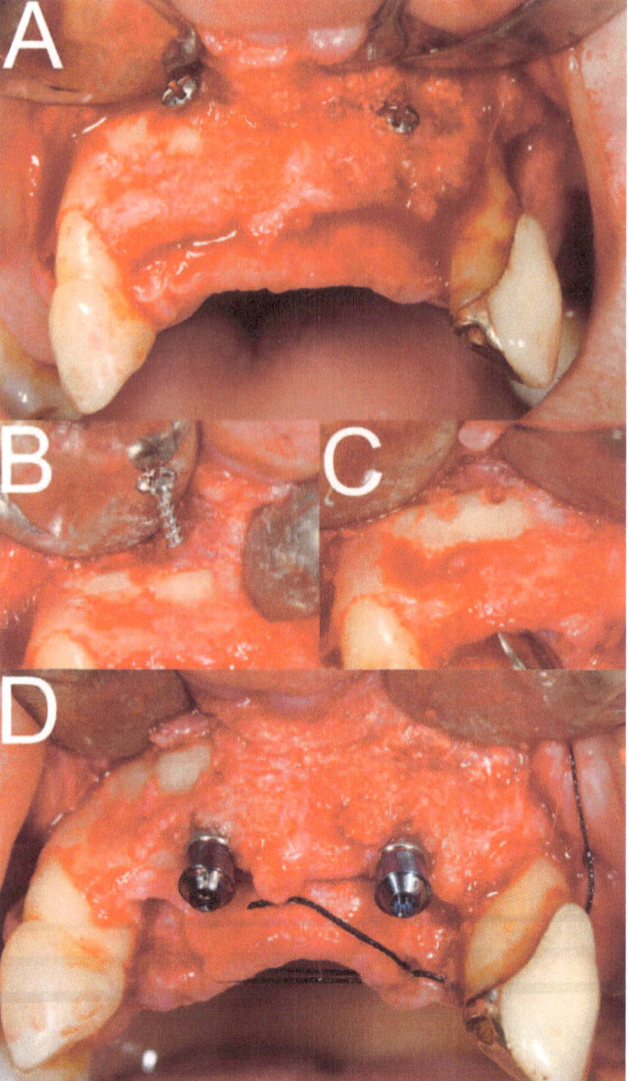

Figure 6-4. *Implant surgery of the case depicted in Figures 6-1, 6-2 and 6-3. A) Clinical view of the grafted anterior maxilla after a six-month healing period. B) Fixation screws were released. C) Aspect of the osseointegrated block grafts D) Two Straumann® Bone Level implants (3.3 x 10 mm) were installed to rehabilitate the case.*

In order to achieve success with onlay bone graft procedures, the shape of the blocks should be carefully adjusted to optimize contact with the recipient site and to obtain an adequate bone contour of the reconstructed alveolar ridge. Careful assessment of both recipient and donor sites using CBCT is also a prerequisite to conduct treatment planning. For this purpose, linear and volumetric measurement tools are available on the interface of DICOM viewers. Onlay blocks have to be firmly secured to the recipient bone surfaces with screws made of either titanium or a resorbable biomaterial. Regardless of the screw type, fixation screw sites should also be determined and measured in 3D multiplanar reconstructions from CBCT scans. Titanium screws are stronger, but need to be removed before implant placement, sometimes resulting in screw fracture during the procedure. Resorbable screws are weaker but do not need to be removed. Both screw systems offer predictable clinical results.[19] As the screws are tightened, the cancellous portion of the allogeneic block is compressed, decreasing the spacing at the bone-graft interface to the point that an intimate contact is established between the graft and the host bone. Block compression increases bone density, which favors the migration of osteoblasts and graft revascularization.[20] Furthermore, satisfactory block adaptation has been found to be essential in the prevention of fibrous ingrowth between allografts and host bone. Before suturing, periosteal releasing incisions should also be performed to allow for tension-free closure of the flaps.

Although onlay bone grafts are frequently placed without the use of barrier membranes to take advantage of the vascular supply provided from the periosteum, recent studies have tested the benefits of covering onlay bone grafts with resorbable membranes (Figure 6-5). This procedure has been shown to be beneficial in preventing bone graft resorption due to masticatory forces.[10] However, there are insufficient evidences of the efficacy of barrier membranes as responsible to prevent the resorption of onlay bone grafts. Risk of membrane exposure during the healing period and subsequent complications should also be considered.

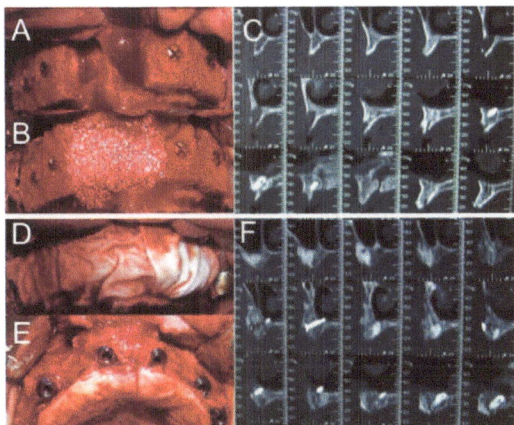

Figure 6-5. Onlay grafts with barrier membranes. A) Clinical view of a patient in which a cancellous block

graft surgery was performed in anterior region. B) All gaps between grafts were filled with anorganic bovine bone (Bio-Oss®, Geistlich AG, Wolhusen, Switzerland). C) CT cross-sectional images of the patient showing several bone defects preventing implant placement. D) Membranes were used to cover all cancellous block grafts. E) Clinical view of the patient 4 months after surgery showing significant resorption despite the use of membranes. However, the remaining bone was sufficient for implants placement. F) CT images 4 months after surgery showing the horizontal bone augmentation achieved, although discrete graft resorption could also be observed.

In contrast, there are studies suggesting that the periosteum contributes to early revascularization and prevention of bone resorption.[21] Recent research has suggested that periosteal preservation is as effective as a barrier membrane in protecting combined particulate/block grafts in large size defects.[22] In addition, the use of pericranium as an autogenous membrane for covering onlay bone grafts in the reconstruction of the atrophic maxilla has been found to reduce the incidence of soft tissue dehiscences and subsequent graft resorption.[13] The use of autogenous block bone grafts in combination with anorganic bovine bone has also been suggested as useful to avoid bone resorption. Another option proposed to ensure graft healing and minimize their resorption is to cover the blocks with platelet-rich plasma (PRP).[17]

There are two types of autografts: cancellous or cortical. Cancellous autografts are considered the gold-standard graft. It leads to fast revascularization due to the activity of mesenchymal cells (osteoblasts precursors) present in the bone marrow, which have the capacity to survive and proliferate after exposure to changes in the oxygen tension, pH and cytochine environment.

Cortical autografts are segments of cortical bone that provides an osteoconductive support for bone formation. However, it does not have significant amounts of important living cells. For this reason, revascularization and osseointegration of cortical autografts occur slowly. The main advantage of cortical autografts is the compressive strength and mechanical support that is provided at the graft site.[7] Incorporation is initiated by osteoclasts instead of osteoblasts and an extensive resorption may occur in around two weeks after surgery, increasing until about six months; thereafter, the rate of resorption gradually declines to regular levels at one year. Nevertheless it is recommended to wait at least four months for graft healing and incorporation to perform implant placement.

Bone Xenografts

Bone xenograft is one the most researched types of block grafts in studies on oral rehabilitation. Bone xenograft is defined as a bone tissue harvested from one species and implanted into a different species (Figures 6-6 and 6-7). One of the most commonly used xenografts is anorganic bovine bone (ABB). ABB is a biomaterial with short- and long-term success reports described in the literature on bone regeneration.[6]

The structural composition of ABB is similar to the human bone. It is basically composed of almost pure hydroxyapatite, and it is chemically treated to remove all organic components so that it does not cause host immune response. ABB is thermally and chemically treated in order to extract its organic constituents and thereby minimizing the potential inflammatory response by the host bone. The structure consists of a wide interconnective pore system with particle sizes ranging from 0.25 to 1 mm, and it is easily penetrated by blood vessels, which results in osteoblastic migration. ABB is up to 75% porous and has a large surface area that results in increased angiogenesis and newly formed bone growth enhancement,[23] with good osteoconduction properties. However, its high porous consistency may also compromise its mechanical properties and its initial stability. ABB lacks osteoinductive properties, and its common presentation in form of granules makes it difficult to be stable on surgical sites. Moreover, ABB might need several years (3-6 years) of implantation before being significantly resorbed by osteoclast activity. Skoglung and collaborators[24] reported that granules are present even 44 months after the grafting procedure. The presence of graft granules within areas of new bone formation is undesired because it affects the quality of the newly formed bone by interfering with its remodeling process.

Although ABB is mostly used in form of granules, xenografts blocks are also available. Xenogeneic derived bone blocks have already been reported as an option to achieve vertical bone augmentation.

However, their structure is fragile. This mechanical inconvenience not only complicates the surgical technique but also hinders the bone graft healing process.[25] Other types of xenogeneic (porcine) bone block seem to show better mechanical properties and low risk of fracture while screwing. However, the use of xenogeneic bone blocks is currently under evaluation and there is still no sufficient information regarding its *in vivo* behavior. One of the few evidences was described by a study from Pistilli and collaborators,[26] who conducted a pilot randomized controlled trial between AB and Xenografts. This study indicated that results from autogenous onlay bone blocks are clearly superior to equine onlay bone blocks, especially in the mandible, where all equine blocks failed. As a result, the authors suggest that the use of onlay bone blocks of equine origin in mandibles should be avoided.[26]

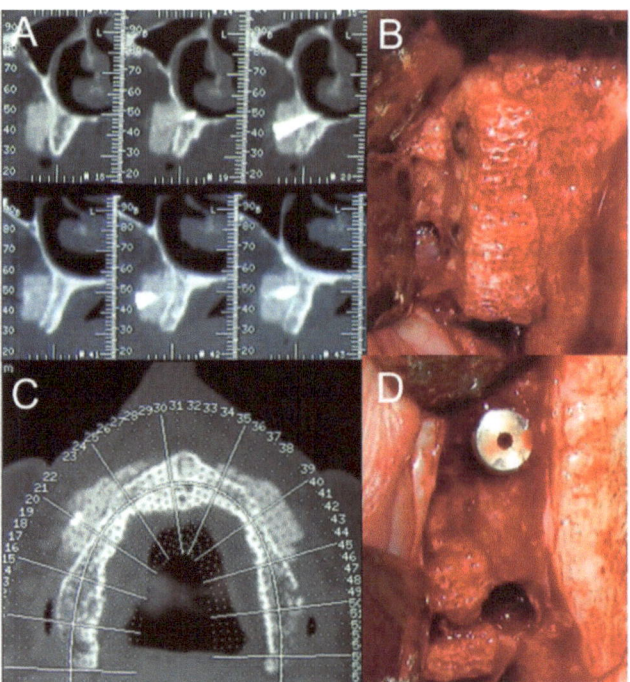

Figure 6-6. *Porcine xenograft blocks A) CT scan of a horizontal bone augmentation, showing satisfactory volume with four months after surgery. B) Clinical view before removal of the fixation screws. C) Axial CT image showing the extension of horizontal bone augmentation achieved. D) Block detachment during implant drilling due to lack of incorporation.*

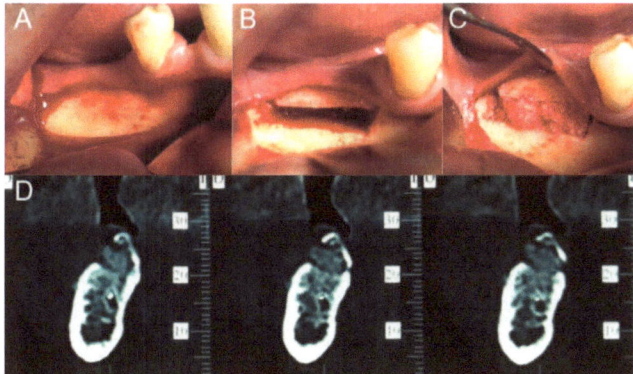

Figure 6-7. *The use of a porcine xenograft block graft in the sandwich technique. A) Buccal flap B) Horizontal and vertical osteotomy was performed with piezoelectric surgery. The superior segment was moved upward and raised to the level of the alveolar crest. C) Clinical aspect of the interpositional porcine block. Particulate anorganic bovine bone was used to fill the existing gaps. D) CT scan taken four months after grafting procedure showing vertical augmentation.*

Allografts

Allograft is defined as a tissue that has been harvested from one individual and implanted into another individual of the same species.[21] The use of cadaver bone as allografts is considered one of the best available alternatives to autografts, due its similar biologic characteristics. Despite the superior properties of autografts, allografts are usually preferred by patients to avoid problems associated to bone harvesting. Allografts can be obtained at cadaver tissue banks usually from cortical areas of long bones due to its higher content of bone inductive proteins and lower antigenic activity, as compared to cancellous bone. Bone allografts are offered in various configurations, including powder, cortical chips, cancellous cubes, and cortical and cancellous granules.[21] Moreover, allografts are also available in different block forms, although their mechanical properties are slightly worse than those of autograft cortical blocks.

Cases of disease transmission as a result of allograft transplant have been reported in the past, when obsolete donor screening procedures were used. Nevertheless, new screening protocols have significantly increased the procedure safety, thus minimizing risks. Once the allograft is harvested they are processed through several methods including physical debridement to remove soft tissue and ultrasonic washing to remove remnant cells. Blood ethanol treatment is also carried out to denaturalize proteins and viral deactivation. The procedure also includes antibiotic wash and sterilization through gamma radiation and ethylene oxide for spore elimination). The main ways to preserve bone are fresh-freezing and freeze-drying. Deep-frozen bone, whether irradiated or not, retains most of its original mechanical properties. In the frozen state, damage to collagen is reduced because of the smaller amounts of free radicals generated by ionization of frozen water, whereas at room temperature, more free radicals are produced.

In the preparation of freeze-dried materials, most of the water content is usually removed. However, this procedure involves ionization that leads to scission of the collagen chains, which in turn may compromise the mechanical resistance of the graft. For this reason, it is advised to rehydrate allografts before using to regain some of the lost properties.[27] Freeze-dried and sterilized bone can provide mechanical stability under compression, but because of its low resistance, this type of bone should be used in an area that is mechanically protected.

Processed bone allografts do not include any living cells, and therefore lack osteogeneic activity. On the other hand, allografts provide satisfactory osteoconduction. However, since mineralized bone matrix has no active bone morphogenetic proteins (BMPs), allografts lack osteoinductive properties.

Allograft incorporation is qualitatively similar to autografts, but occurs more slowly. The main advantages of allografts are higher availability, avoiding the need of harvesting a patient donor site; higher patient's acceptance, reduced costs in terms of anesthesia (general anesthesia is not needed) and reduced surgical time. Although block allografts were introduced four decades ago, they have only recently been studied and used as onlays for alveolar bone augmentation, proving useful in both vertical and horizontal bone augmentation procedures.[28,29]

Although some studies reported immunological reactions using some types of allografts freeze-dried allografts are unlikely to induce sensitization response in the host tissue. Freeze-dried allografts are the most commonly used grafting material for interbody fusion of the cervical, thoracic, and lumbar spines. In implant dentistry, however, the most frequently reported type of block allograft in studies is the fresh frozen one, especially in the form of cortico-cancellous blocks, which combine the properties of both cancellous bone that allows vascular infiltration, and cortical bone that provides rigid fixation and mechanical resistance.

Clinical studies have suggested that predictable results can be obtained with implants placed in bone augmented with allograft onlays, achieving a success rate over 90% after at least one-year follow-up.[30-32] Further studies would still be recommended to address long-term success rates of implants placed in the bone augmented with allografts.

Cancellous allograft block

There is little information regarding the use of cancellous allograft bone block in implant dentistry. However, it has been described that successful long-term results can be achieved. One of the studies showed an implant survival rate of 95% in a mean 30-month follow-up.[30] Although allograft remodeling and revascularization properties are significantly inferior compared with fresh autogenous bone graft, Nissan and collaborators[31] observed a rate of 33% of new bone formation using allografts, with an implant survival rate of 98% in a mean 48-month follow-up. The authors of the aforementioned study also observed that new bone formation rate was age-dependent. This study concluded that cancellous bone block allograft (Figure 6-8) is biocompatible and osteoconductive, enabling new bone formation following onlay augmentation of extremely atrophic anterior maxilla.[31]

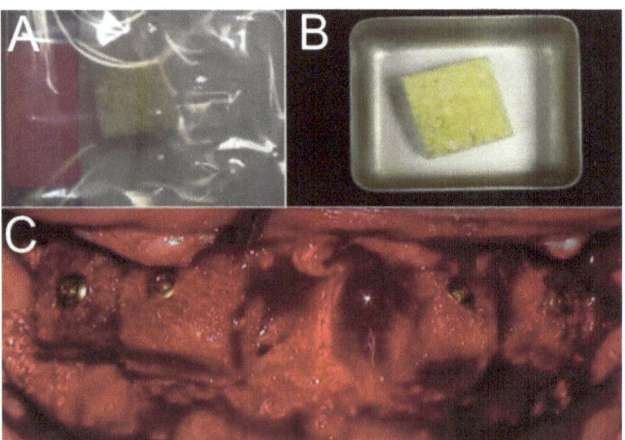

Figure 6-8. *Cancellous allograft block (Tutogen Medical Gmbh, Neunkirchen, Germany). A) Presentation. B) Block preparing. C) Blocks used to rehabilitate an atrophic maxilla.*

Cortico-Cancellous allograft block

Despite controversial results previously described in the literature, Peleg and collaborators[20] presented encouraging clinical findings using onlay cortico-cancellous grafts. In this study, of a total of 57 block grafts placed, only one showed a minimal area of resorption, which did not prevent placement of dental implants in appropriate positions. Moreover, of the total of 84 implants placed, only one failed to osseointegrate. Despite the relatively short follow-up period, the authors suggest that cortico-cancellous allogeneic bone block grafts (Figure 6-9) are a viable alternative to autogenous bone block grafts in patients with alveolar ridge deficiencies.[20] However, there is only a few controlled long-term follow-up studies confirming the above-mentioned findings.

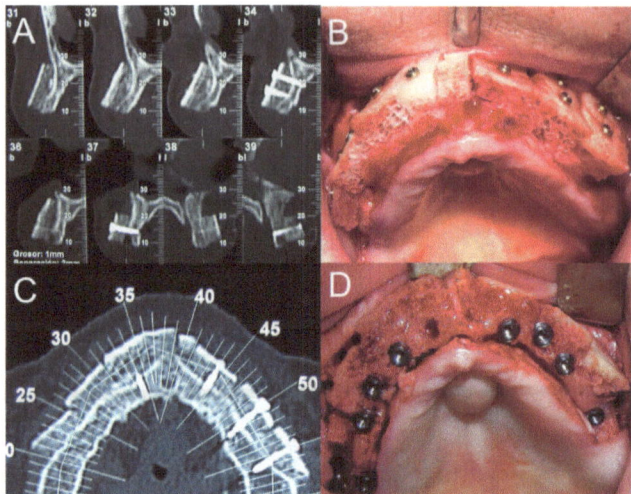

Figure 6-9. *Cortico-cancellous allograft. A) CBCT Cross-sectional image taken four months after block surgery, (the buccal plate maintained its original position and the total volume did not undergo significant changes). B) Blocks stabilized with screws. C) CBCT Axial image taken four months after block surgery showing good conditions of the blocks. D) Clinical view of the implants placed in the augmented area, where no significant resorption could be observed.*

Early bone resorption

Early resorptions can be considered as those that take place from the moment of graft surgery to a 6-month follow-up, which is an adequate healing time for auto- and allografts. One of the most common clinical signs indicating early resorptions is the presence of soft tissue dehiscences. In this context, block allografts are more technique sensitive than autografts, and usually require a more meticulous surgical technique. The type and density of bone in relation to its architecture may also have an impact on bone resorption. Furthermore, cancellous block grafts usually present significant higher resorption rates, as compared with cortico-cancellous bone blocks, in a 4-month observation period (Figure 6-10).

Late bone resorption

Late resorptions are those that take place during a follow-up period from 1 to 5 years. In late resoptions, the type and density of bone are probably the most determinant factors. In this context, autografts present lower resorption rates than allografts. Furthermore, the embryologic origin of an autograft may also have influence on resorption rates. It has been confirmed that better results can be achieved with intramembranous sources, as compared with endochondral sources. A study based on CT observations revealed that both autografts and allografts might undergo extensive resorption at 6 months. However, in their results, cases with allografts lost significantly more bone volume.[22] The larger resorption of the allografs grafts (Figure 6-11) can probably be attributed to an inadequate revascularization, less bone ingrowth inside the grafted block, and/or a smaller number of cells involved in the remodelling process of this type of bone graft.[33] Early vascularization of the graft is a main factor contributing to the integration of the graft and the maintenance of its stability. Vascular invasion has been noted at one week after allograft placement, and permeation of the entire graft occurs by the 3- to 6-week period. However, vascularization and new intramembranous bone deposition rates observed with allografts at 12 weeks will only be similar to the ones obtained with autografts at the 3- to 6-week evaluation.[20]

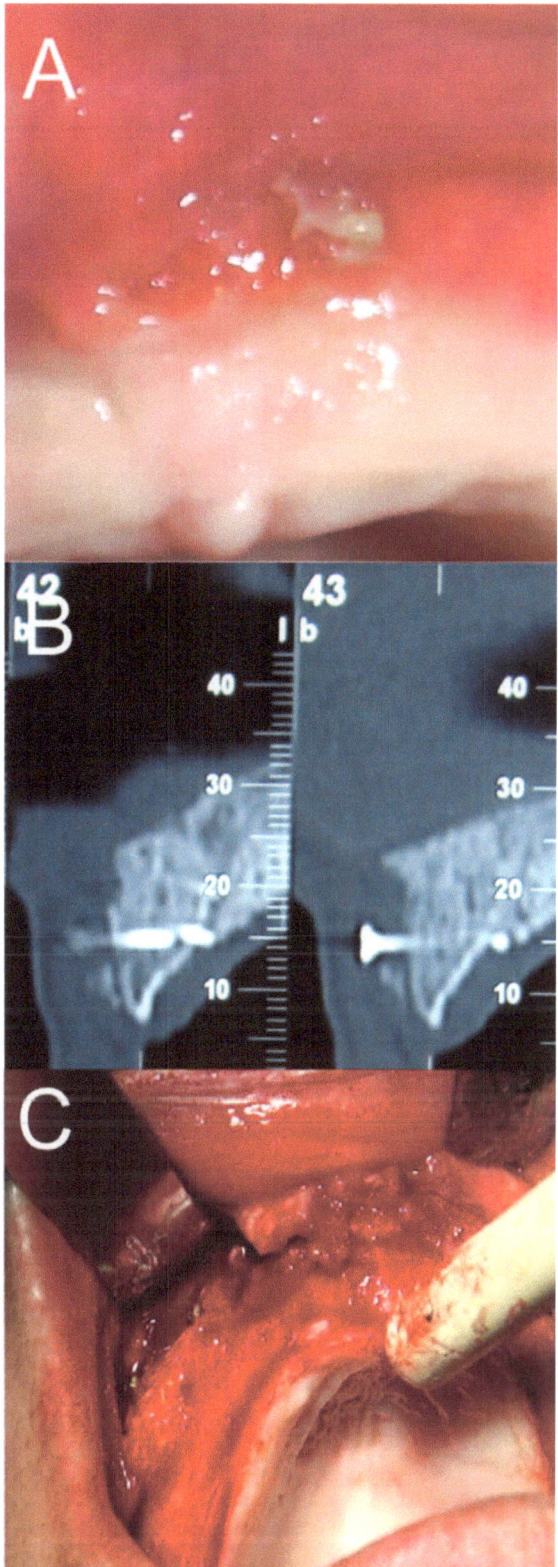

Figure 6-10. Early block bone resorption. A) Clinical sign of soft tissue dehiscence. B) CBCT cross-sectional image showing significant resorption. C) Clinical view showing area with graft resorption.

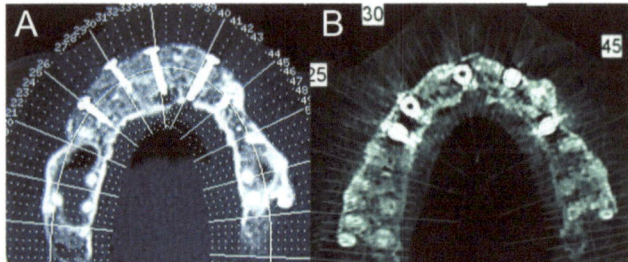

Figure 6-11. *Late block bone resorption. A) CT axial image taken four months after cancellous block allograft surgery, which allowed for the placement of five implants in the anterior region. B) Five-year follow-up image showing significant resorption, although implants remained in satisfactory conditions.*

A study on bone graft incorporation found relatively poorer results of vital bone formation with allografs, in comparison with autografts, observed 6 months after the grafting procedure.[28] In contrast, Lumetti and collaborators[22] observed no significant differences between autogenous and allogeneic bone block grafts regarding percentages of newly formed vital bone at the same study time. Incorporation of a graft within the host bone depends not only on the type of graft but also on the conditions of the bone at the site of the transplant, quality of the transplanted bone and of the host bone, host site preparation, graft preservation techniques, systemic and local health conditions, and mechanical properties of the graft.

Synthetic calcium phosphate
The group of calcium phosphates includes synthetic biomaterials that chemically resemble the bone mineral. Calcium phosphate biomaterials are widely used as bone graft substitutes due to their biocompatibility and osteoconductivity.[4,5]

Hydroxyapatite and β-tricalcium phosphate (β-TCP) are among the most recruited materials to treat bone defects. These ceramics are presented in porous granular and block forms. In addition, new synthetic bone substitutes have been developed to eliminate the need of autologous grafts and to overcome their limitations. Among these materials, dicalcium phosphate anhydrous (monetite) is of special interest because it is a biocompatible, resorbable, osteoconductive and osteoinductive biomaterial.[34]

Monetite onlays could be suitable for vertical bone augmentation, and can be produced in customized designs using 3D-printing. Dental implants can be successfully placed in onlays with the newly formed bone occupying 30-40% of its total volume. In addition, monetite onlays used for vertical bone augmentation could be infiltrated by new bone *in vivo*, occupying up to 43% of the graft volume after 8 weeks implantation.[34] So far, however, there are no *in vivo* evidences of satisfactory results from any synthetic alternative to onlay autogenous bone grafts for alveolar ridge augmentation in humans.

References

1. Jang HY, Kim HC, Lee SC, Lee JY. Choice of graft material in relation to maxillary sinus width in internal sinus floor augmentation. J Oral Maxillofac Surg 68:1859, 2010.

2. Smiler DG. The sinus lift graft: basic technique and variations. Pract Periodontics Aesthet Dent 9:885, 1997.

3. Schlegel K.A, Fichtner G, Schultze-Mosgau S, Wiltfang J. Histologic findings in sinus augmentation with autogenous bone chips versus a bovine bone substitute. Int J Oral Maxillofac Implants 18:53, 2003.

4. Tosta M, Cortes AR, Corrêa L, Pinto Junior DS, Tumenas I, Katchburian E. Histologic and histomorphometric evaluation of a synthetic bone substitute for maxillary sinus grafting in humans. Clin Oral Implants Res 2013;24:866-70.

5. Cortes AR, Cortes DN, Arita ES. Correction of buccal dehiscence at the time of implant placement without using barrier membranes: A retrospective cone beam computed tomographic study. Int J Oral Maxillofac Implants 2013;28:1564-9.

6. Cortes AR, Corrêa L, Arita ES. Evaluation of a Maxillary Sinus Floor Augmentation in the Presence of a Large Antral Pseudocyst. J Craniofac Surg 2012;23:e535-7.

7. Bauer TW, Muschler GF. Bone graft materials. An overview of the basic science. Clin Orthop Relat Res. 2000 Feb;(371):10-27.

8. Triplett RG, Schow SR. Autologous bone grafts and endosseous implants: Complementary techniques. J Oral Maxillofac Surg 1996;54:486-94.

9. Aghaloo TL, Moy PK. Which hard tissue augmentation techniques are the most successful in

furnishing bony support for implant placement? Int J Oral Maxillofac Implants 2007;22(suppl):49-70.

10. Rocchietta I, Fontana F, Simion M. Clinical outcomes of vertical bone augmentation to enable dental implant placement: a systematic review. J Clin Periodontol 2008;35(Suppl.8):203–15.

11. Li J, Wang HL. Common implant-related advanced bone grafting complications: classification, etiology, and management. Implant Dent 2008;17:389-401.

12. Sjöström M, Sennerby L, Nilson H, et al. Reconstruction of the atrophic edentulous maxilla with free iliac crest grafts and implants: A 3-year report of a prospective clinical study. Clin Implant Dent Relat Res 2007;9:46-59.

13. Chiapasco M, Zaniboni M, Boisco M. Augmentation procedures for the rehabilitation of deficient edentulous ridges with oral implants. Clin Oral Implants Res 2006;17(Suppl.2):136-59.

14. Chiapasco M, Zaniboni M, Rimondini L. Autogenous onlay bone grafts vs. alveolar distraction osteogenesis for the correction of vertically deficient edentulous ridges: a 2-4-year prospective study on humans. Clin Oral Implants Res 2007;18(4):432-40.

15. Tamura K, Sato S, Kishida M, Asano S, Murai M, Ito K. The use of porous beta-tricalcium phosphate blocks with platelet-rich plasma as an onlay bone graft biomaterial. J Periodontol 2007;78(2):315-21.

16. Tamimi F, Torres J, Gbureck U, Lopez-Cabarcos E, Bassett DC, Alkhraisat MH, Barralet JE. Craniofacial vertical bone augmentation: a comparison between 3D printed monolithic monetite blocks and autologous onlay grafts in the rabbit. Biomaterials 2009;30(31):6318-26.

17. Torres J, Tamimi F, Alkhraisat MH, Manchón A, Linares R, Prados-Frutos JC, Hernández G, López Cabarcos E. Platelet-rich plasma may prevent titanium-mesh exposure in alveolar ridge augmentation with anorganic bovine bone. J Clin Periodontol 2010;37(10):943-51.

18. Waasdorp J, Reynolds MA. Allogeneic bone onlay grafts for alveolar ridge augmentation: a systematic review. Int J Oral Maxillofac Implants 2010;25(3):525-31.

19. Quereshy FA, Dhaliwal HS, El SA, Horan MP, Dhaliwal SS. Resorbable screw fixation for cortical onlay bone grafting: a pilot study with preliminary results. J Oral Maxillofac Surg 2010;68(10):2497-502.

20. Peleg M, Sawatari Y, Marx RN, Santoro J, Cohen J, Bejarano P, Malinin T. Use of corticocancellous allogeneic bone blocks for augmentation of alveolar bone defects. Int J Oral Maxillofac Implants 2010;25(1):153-62.

21. Park KD, Hong H, Jung S, Kook MS, Oh HK, Park H. Effect of periosteum attached to autogenous iliac block bone graft on bone resorption in rabbits. J Craniofac Surg 2015;26(3):642-6.

22. Verdugo F, D'Addona A, Pontón J. Clinical, tomographic, and histological assessment of periosteal guided bone regeneration with cortical perforations in advanced human critical size defects. Clin Implant Dent Relat Res 2012;14(1):112-20

21. Eppley BL, Pietrzak WS, Blanton MW: Allograft and alloplastic bone substitutes: A review of science and technology for the craniomaxillofacial surgeon. J Craniofac Surg 2005;16:981-9.

22. Lumetti S, Consolo U, Galli C, Multinu A, Piersanti L, Bellini P, Manfredi E, Corinaldesi G, Zaffe D, Macaluso GM, Marchetti C. Fresh-frozen bone blocks for horizontal ridge augmentation in the upper maxilla: 6-month outcomes of a randomized controlled trial. Clin Implant Dent Relat Res 2014;16(1):116-23.

23. Hämmerle CH, Olah AJ, Schmid J, Flückiger L, Gogolewski S, Winkler JR, Lang NP. The biological effect of natural bone mineral on bone neoformation on the rabbit skull. Clin Oral Implants Res 1997;8(3):198-207.

24. Skoglund A, Hising P, Young C. A clinical and histologic examination in humans of the osseous response to implanted natural bone mineral. Int J Oral Maxillofac Implants 1997;12(2):194-9.

25. Simion M, Rocchietta I, Kim D, Nevins M, Fiorellini J. Vertical ridge augmentation by means of deproteinized bovine bone block and recombinant human platelet-derived growth factor-BB: a histologic study in a dog model. Int J Periodontics Restorative Dent. 2006 Oct;26(5):415-23.

26. Pistilli R, Felice P, Piatelli M, Nisii A, Barausse C, Esposito M. Blocks of autogenous bone versus xenografts for the rehabilitation of atrophic jaws with dental implants: preliminary data from a pilot randomised controlled trial. Eur J Oral Implantol. 2014;7(2):153-71.

27. Kao ST, Scott DD. A review of bone substitutes. ral Maxillofac Surg Clin North Am 2007;19(4):513-21

28. Spin-Neto R, Stavropoulos A, Coletti FL, Faeda RS, Pereira LA, Marcantonio E Jr. Graft incorporation

and implant osseointegration following the use of autologous and fresh-frozen allogeneic block bone grafts for lateral ridge augmentation. Clin Oral Implants Res 2014;25:226-33.

29. Al-Abedalla K, Torres J, Cortes AR, Wu X, Nader SA, Daniel N, Tamimi F. Bone Augmented With Allograft Onlays for Implant Placement Could Be Comparable With Native Bone. J Oral Maxillofac Surg. 2015 Jun 20. pii: S0278-2391(15)00819-8.

30. Nissan J, Mardinger O, Strauss M, Peleg M, Sacco R, Chaushu G. Implant-supported restoration of congenitally missing teeth using cancellous bone block-allografts. Oral Surg Oral Med Oral Pathol Oral Radiol Endod 2011;111:286-91.

31. Nissan J, Marilena V, Gross O, Mardinger O, Chaushu G. Histomorphometric analysis following augmentation of the anterior atrophic maxilla with cancellous bone block allograft. Int J Oral Maxillofac Implants 2012;27:84-9

32. Novell J, Novell-Costa F, Ivorra C, Fariñas O, Munilla A, Martinez C. Five-year results of implants inserted into freeze-dried block allografts. Implant Dent 2012;21:129-35.

33. Goldberg VM, Stevenson S. Natural history of autografts and allografts. Clin Orthop Relat Res 1987;(225):7-16.

34. Tamimi F, Torres J, Al-Abedalla K, Lopez-Cabarcos E, Alkhraisat MH, Bassett DC, Gbureck U, Barralet JE. Osseointegration of dental implants in 3D-printed synthetic onlay grafts customized according to bone metabolic activity in recipient site. Biomaterials. 2014 Jul;35(21):5436-45.

CHAPTER 7

SINUS FLOOR AUGMENTATION

Arthur Rodriguez Gonzalez Cortes
Djalma Nogueira Cortes

Maxillary sinuses are air-filled cavities that usually develop symmetrically in the bones of the face. Although their function is not completely clear, some features such as reduction of the skull weight and mucus production have been described.

The maxillary sinus has a pyramidal shape with its base corresponding to the lateral wall of the nasal cavity and its apex corresponding to the zygomatic bone. The maxillary sinus roof corresponds to the floor of the orbital cavity, while the sinus anterior wall corresponds to the facial surface of the maxilla. The posterior bone wall of the maxillary sinus separates it from two anatomical structures: the pterygomaxillary fossa (medially) and the infratemporal fossa (laterally). The most lateral extension of the maxillary sinus is the zygomatic recess. Medially, the maxillary sinus has an ostium, which drains into the nasal cavity through the infundibulum. The maxillary sinus floor is formed by the hard palate and the alveolar process of the maxillary bone.

Sinus floor augmentation

The increasing number of researches on oral implantology led to the establishment of various bone grafting techniques for overcoming bone loss and improving the success of dental implant therapy in cases with severely resorbed maxilla.[1-5] Maxillary sinus floor grafting can be performed with different techniques, such as the osteotome internal sinus-lift procedure and the lateral window approach. This, in turn, is a predictable way of achieving sufficient bone height for posterior maxillary implant placement.[6-10]

Usually, the aim of maxillary sinus augmentation is to obtain a final ridge height of at least 10 mm, allowing the placement of endosseous dental implants. Nevertheless, some intrasurgical and postoperative complications may compromise surgical outcomes and even lead to implant loss.[11]

The most common surgical complication is the perforation of the Schneiderian membrane. It occurs in 14% to 56% of sinus lift procedures, usually during the lateral window preparation or during curet elevation of the membrane.[6,7]

Piezoelectric surgery

Piezoelectric surgery is an option to potentially reduce the risk of sinus lift surgical complications, including Schneiderian membrane perforation.[12,13] The use of a piezoelectric surgical unit has been described as a technological method, useful to perform precise osteotomies in different types of grafting surgeries.[12,13] The issue of the close relationship of hard to soft tissues in the maxillary sinus is solved by this method as it does not cut soft tissues. As a result, it is reasonable to assume that proper piezoelectric use in the preparation of lateral sinus antrostomies should decrease the risk of intrasurgical complications, such as Schneiderian membrane perforation and sinus arterial lacerations, even in cases of very thin sinus bone walls or of septa presence.[13,14] For additional safety, angles of a rectangular osteotomy should be rounded and softened, so as to minimize the risk of injuring the membrane.

Anatomical variations of the maxillary sinus

Anatomical aspects of the maxillary sinus such as sinus antrum dimensions, presence of septa, as well as thickness of sinus bone walls and of the Schneiderian membrane, vary from one patient to the other.[3] Moreover, maxillary edentulism, oral and maxillofacial pathologies, and previous surgeries are considered factors that can alter the maxillary sinus anatomy.[3,15] Normally, the average dimensions of an adult sinus are 2.5 to 3.5 cm in width, 3.6 to 4.5 cm in height, and 3.8 to 4.5 cm in length, and the sinus membrane has a thickness of approximately 1 mm.[15] Sinus anatomical conditions, such as septa (Figures 7-1 and 7-2) or a thin membrane, have been indicated as factors that increase the risk of Schneiderian membrane perforation.[15,16] In this context, CBCT images are useful for obtaining detailed information on the maxillary sinus for surgical planning and postoperative evaluation.[17] The impact of these anatomical variations on sinus lifting surgeries has been addressed by some articles in the literature.

A study on the lateral window approach, described the rate of occurrence of anatomical variations of the sinus bone walls, size, and membrane (Table 7-1).[18]

Table 7-1. Frequency of occurrence of anatomical alterations reported in the literature[18] and impact on sinus membrane perforation during sinus floor augmentation with the lateral window approach.

Sinus anatomical variations	%	Risk of sinus membrane perforation
Antral septa	32.5%	Low
Narrow antrum	55%	Low
Very thin bone wall	72.5%	Low
Very thin membrane	62.5%	Medium
Scars/Previous operations	7.5%	Medium-High
Failure in the sinus floor bone	2.5%	Medium (if it is small) and High (if it is large)

Presence of antral septa and failure in sinus floor bone can be detected by preoperative CBCT images. Linear, area and volumetric measurements can also be performed in the 3D CBCT multiplanar reconstructions to detect narrow sinus antrum (less than 25mm in width), very thin lateral bone wall or very thin Schneiderian membrane (less than 0.5mm thick). Most of these measurements can be performed by virtual implant planning softwares. However, scars in the Schneiderian membrane can only be detected during the surgical procedure.

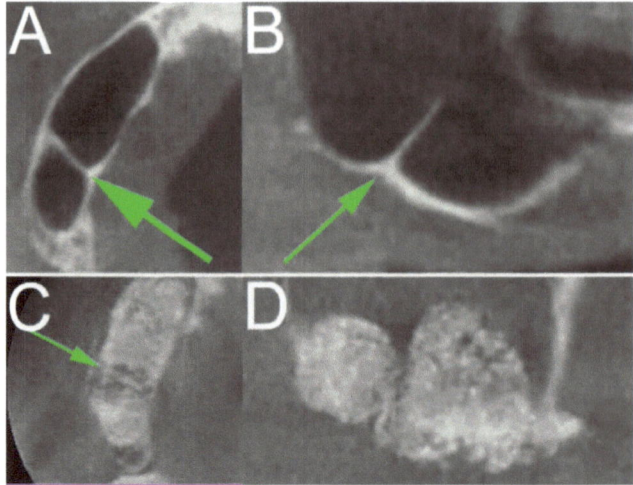

Figure 7-1. CBCT of a sinus bony septum (green arrow). A) Preoperative axial view. B) Preoperative sagittal view. C) Postoperative axial view. D) Postoperative sagittal view (note the two different amounts of graft, which were inserted in different lateral windows).

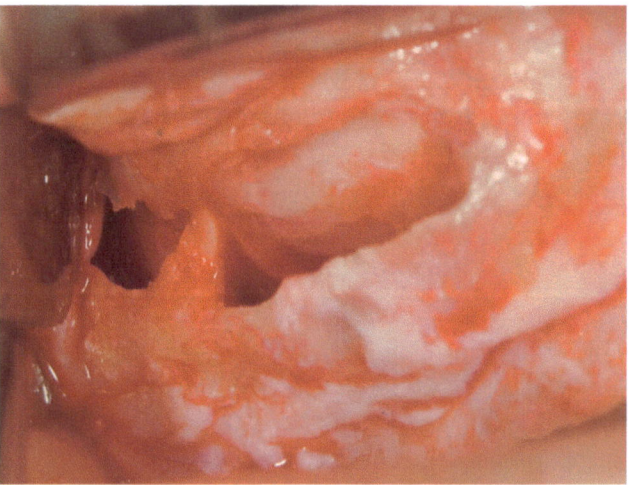

Figure 7-2. Modified lateral window approach to avoid the septum shown in Figure 7-1. Two different lateral windows were created to insert two amounts of graft.

Surgical procedures: imaging considerations

Computed tomographic multiplanar reconstructions are useful to plan and define which is the most appropriate sinus lift surgical technique to be used. Clinical indications for the osteotome technique can be defined during the conventional virtual implant planning. This technique is recommended when more than 6 mm of residual bone height is measured in the cross-sectional image of the implant site. In addition, this technique allows for immediate implant placement, after gaining 3 to 4 mm in bone height.[19]

On the other hand, the lateral window approach can be performed with (one-stage approach) or without immediate implant placement (two-stage approach). One-stage lateral window approaches are indicated in cases with at least 5 mm of residual bone height, provided that primary stability of the implant is achieved. This approach allows for an average gain of 10 mm in bone height. Cases with less than 4-5 mm should be treated with the two-stage approach, which in turn allows for an average gain of 12.7 mm in bone height (Figure 7-2).[19]

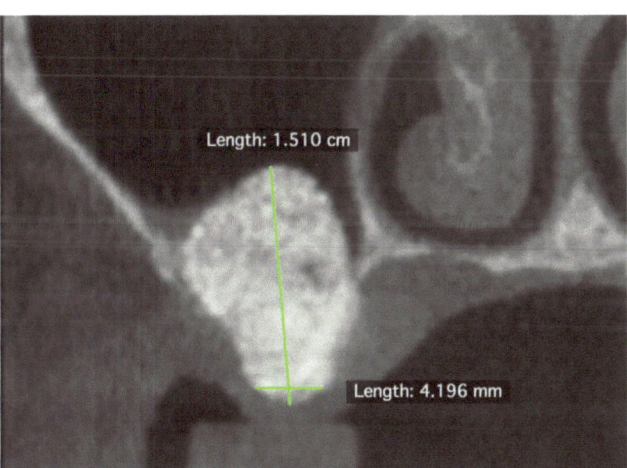

Figure 7-2. CBCT linear measurements in a coronal image of a grafted maxillary sinus.

A series of CT measurements are valuable for planning sinus floor augmentation with the lateral window approach. Linear measurements of the remaining and desired bone width and height can be performed and visualized in 3D reconstructed images. The required volume of sinus graft can also be estimated by using volume measurement tools of radiology softwares (Figure 7-3). Additional linear measurements such as thickness of the lateral bone wall and of the sinus membrane can also be

performed. The angle between the sinus floor and mesial wall (lateral wall of the nasal cavity) should also be assessed, since this is an important angle that should be included in the grafted area (Figure 7-4).

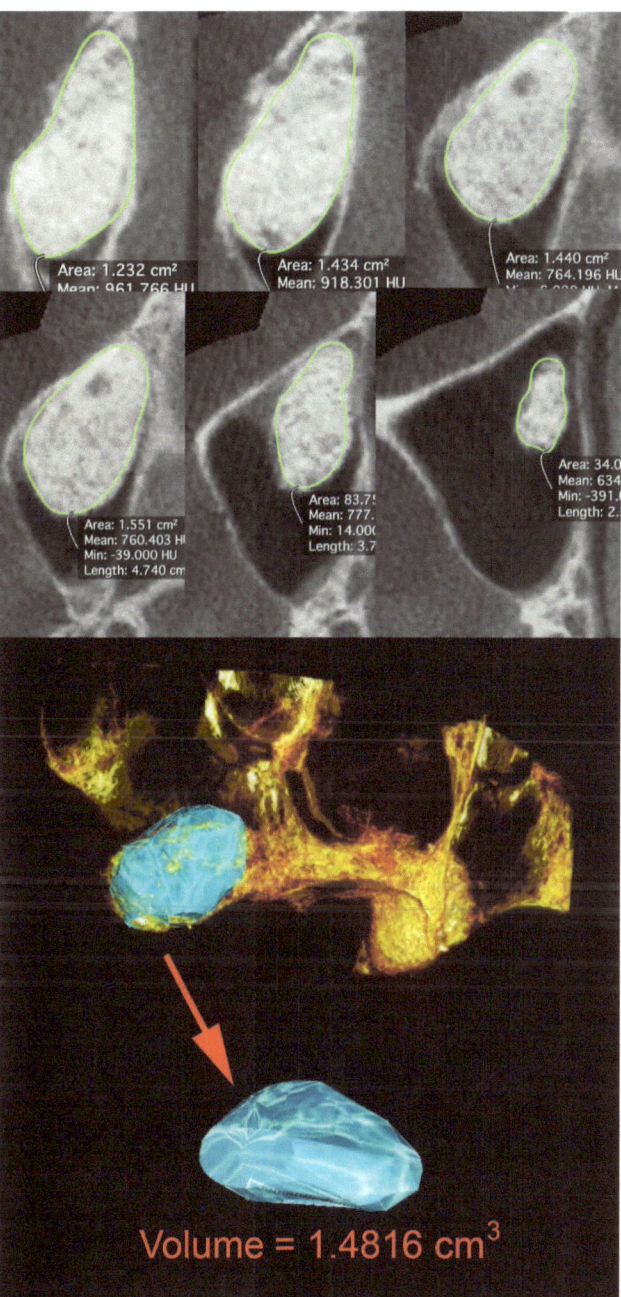

Figure 7-3. CBCT volume measurement of a sinus graft scanned after maturation period. A) The graft area is outlined in all axial slices containing it. B) A 3D ROI is created from the 2D measurements performed in the axial slices with the volumetric measurement tool of the OsiriX software.

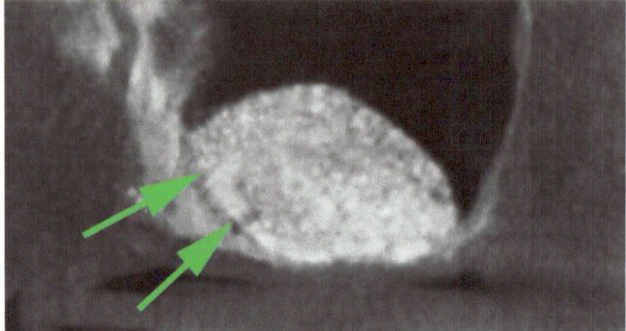

Figure 7-4. *CBCT sagittal view of a grafted maxillary sinus. Note the limit between the graft and the sinus bony wall (green arrows).*

Lateral window approach

The lateral window approach (Figure 7-5) involves elevation of a full-thickness flap that may be initiated slightly palatal to the crest of the ridge. Lateral antrostomy can be created by outlining an island of bone using either a round bur or a piezoelectric unit with a grinding tip. Cooling should always be carried out with a saline solution. In cases presenting antral septa, the lateral window should be performed by outlining to minimize the impact of septa presence. Elevation of the Schneiderian membrane can be performed by initially exposing and mobilizing the membrane using the piezoelectric handpiece with a blunt tip, followed by further elevation of the membrane along the medial wall of the sinus by curet. Grafting materials can then be inserted to perform sinus floor augmentation.

Sinus membrane perforation has been described as one of the most common surgical complications of sinus grafting procedures. It results in a direct communication between the graft material and the contaminated sinus cavity.[20-23] This may cause issues such as infection and chronic sinusitis, which may lead to the loss of graft volume.[20,24,25] Regardless of the effect on outcome parameters, perforations must be repaired so that the graft may be stabilized and the grafting procedure may be completed.[26,27] Membrane repair techniques using bioabsorbable collagen barrier membranes have been reported in the literature and are considered a predictable and safe type of treatment, especially in cases of small perforations.[17,24,25]

As mentioned before, sinus anatomical variations have been described as factors that may increase the risk of membrane perforation.[14,15] The presence of bony septa is considered one of the most common variations related to sinus membrane perforation, and is found in approximately 30% of the sinus lift cases. According to the literature, the incidence of antral septa, especially in younger adults, ranges between 16% and 58%.[4,26] A different osteotomy technique has been described for this situation, consisting in dividing the sinus by preparing two different smaller lateral windows.[4,27,28]

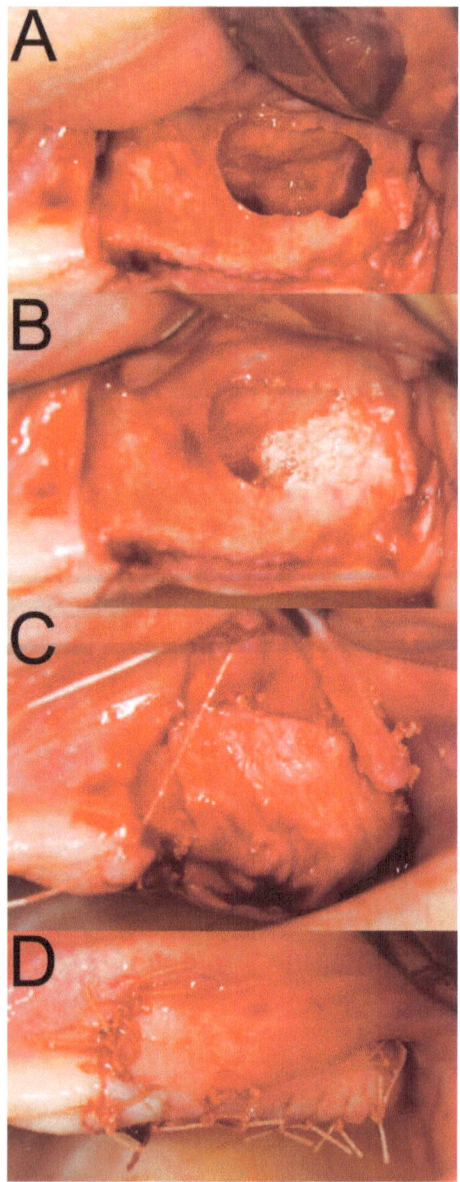

Figure 7-5. *Sinus floor augmentation with the lateral window approach. A) Clinical aspect of the elevated sinus membrane. B) Particulate graft insertion (Straumann BoneCeramic®). C) Collagen Membrane (Geistlich Bio-Gide®, Wolhuser, Switzerland) used to close the window. D) Flaps were secured with vycril sutures.*

Other important factors leading to lower risks of Schneiderian membrane perforation include narrow sinus antrum, very thin sinus bone wall and very thin Schneiderian membranes.[15,24] Scars and signs of a previous operation can even worsen membrane conditions. These types of cases should receive extra care and attention in the surgical planning, so that the sinus floor can be augmented without perforating the sinus membrane.

Antral pseudocysts

Antral pseudocysts are lesions that lack an epithelial lining and are of inflammatory origin, resulting from fluid accumulation within the sinus membrane. Previous studies reported that the presence of an antral cystic lesion could be considered a contraindication for sinus augmentation, and its removal should be performed before undertaking this procedure.[29,30] On the other hand, antral pseudocysts have also been reported not to be contraindicated for sinus floor augmentation procedures when a lateral window approach is used (Figure 7-6).[31,32] In addition, other studies have also suggested the important role played by computed tomography for diagnosing antral pseudocysts and planning sinus grafting surgeries.[33,34] With CBCT scans, it is possible to perform a three-dimensional analysis of the areas with antral pseudocysts and sinus membrane thickening (Figure 7-7). Different CBCT slices and planes can be used to evaluate the extension of the antral pseudocyst area and to evaluate the sinus grafted area, confirming the stability of its position. Additionally, success of graft maturation can be confirmed with histological analysis, which will indicate any presence of inflammatory infiltration in the tissue evaluated.

The most frequently observed differential diagnosis of antral pseudocyst is the sinus mucocele, which has been considered as an extravasation of mucous into adjacent soft tissues. However, their diagnosis includes features such as opacification of the affected sinus and expansion into the adjacent structures. These factors are considered important in differentiating mucoceles, which represent a relative contraindication for sinus lift procedures, from antral pseudocysts.[35]

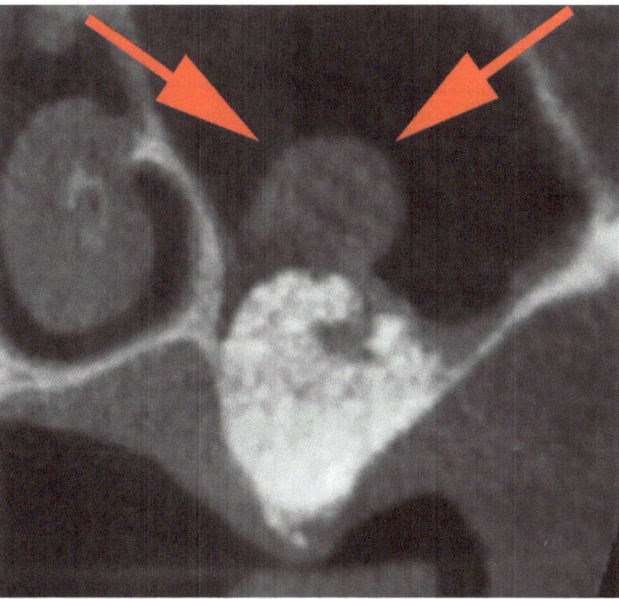

Figure 7-6. *CBCT coronal view of a sinus graft inserted in the presence of an antral pseudocyst (red arrows).*

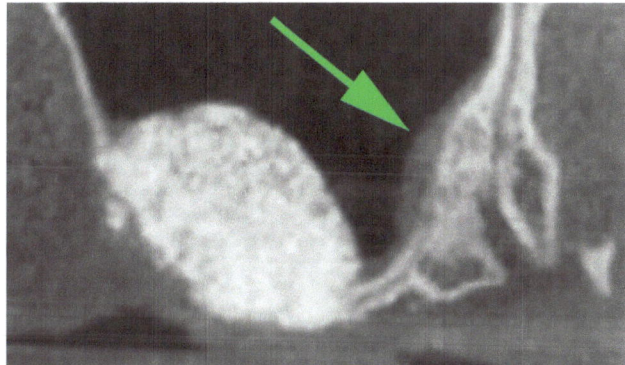

Figure 7-7. *CBCT sagittal view of a sinus graft. Note a slight thickening of the sinus membrane (green arrow).*

Sinus floor failures

Extreme bone resorption in posterior maxilla may lead to absence of part of the sinus floor,[18,36,37] which has been defined as "failure of the sinus floor bone".[18] This is a condition that may compromise sinus floor augmentation. One of the main related complications is that an intimate contact between the Schneiderian membrane and the oral mucosa could occur in the failure areas, thus hindering the surgery from elevating the Schneiderian membrane, and leading to its perforation. CBCT sagittal and coronal images should be used for assessing maxillary sinuses to detect any interruption in the sinus floor bone.[38]

Anatomical alterations of the sinus floor such as convolutions and root-shape expressions, commonly observed in patients with recent teeth extraction, may also cause sinus floor failures and thus render the procedure of elevating the sinus membrane more difficult.[16,17] Sinus floor bone failures (Figure 7-8) were found to be significantly associated with the number of missing posterior teeth and a history of periodontitis, which are factors known to induce bone loss.[38]

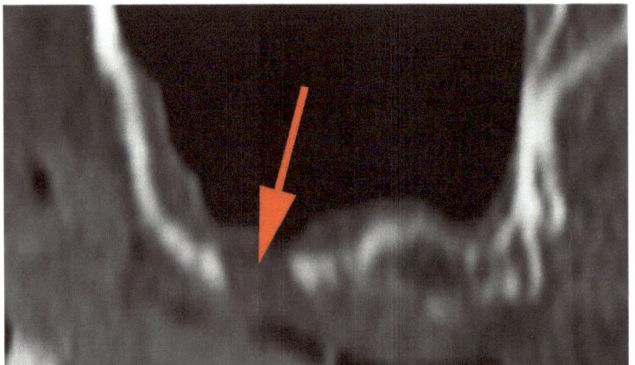

Figure 7-8. CT sagittal view of a sinus floor bone failure (red arrow).

References

1. Boyne PJ, James RA. Grafting of the maxillary sinus floor with autogenous marrow and bone. J Oral Surg 1980;38:613-6.

2. Tatum H Jr. Maxillary and sinus implant reconstructions. Dent Clin North Am 1986;30:207-29.

3. Chanavaz M. Maxillary sinus: anatomy, physiology, surgery, and bone grafting related to implantology--eleven years of surgical experience (1979-1990). J Oral Implantol 1990;16:199-209.

4. Ulm CW, Solar P, Krennmair G, Matejka M, Watzek G. Incidence and suggested surgical management of septa in sinus-lift procedures. Int J Oral Maxillofac Implants 1995 ;10:462-5.

5. Khoury F. Augmentation of the sinus floor with mandibular bone block and simultaneous implantation: a 6-year clinical investigation. Int J Oral Maxillofac Implants 1999;14:557-64.

6. Wallace SS, Froum SJ. Effect of maxillary sinus augmentation on the survival of endosseous dental implants. A systematic review. Ann Periodontol 2003;8:328-43.

7. Del Fabbro M, Testori T, Francetti L, Weinstein R. Systematic review of survival rates for implants placed in the grafted maxillary sinus. Int J Periodontics Restorative Dent 2004;24:565-77.

8. Kaufman E. Maxillary sinus elevation surgery: An overview. J Esthet Restor Dent 2003;15:272-82.

9. Small SA, Zinner ID, Panno FV, Shapiro HJ, Stein JI. Augmenting the maxillary sinus for implants: report of 27 patients. Int J Oral Maxillofac Implants 1993;8:523-8.

10. Kent JN, Block MS. Simultaneous maxillary sinus floor bone grafting and placement of hydroxylapatite-coated implants. J Oral Maxillofac Surg 1989;47:238-42.

11. Fugazzotto PA, Vlassis J. Long-term success of sinus augmentation using various surgical approaches and grafting materials. Int J Oral Maxillofac Implants 1998;13:52-8.

12. Vercellotti T, De Paoli S, Nevins M. The piezoelectric bony window osteotomy and sinus membrane elevation: introduction of a new technique for simplification of the sinus augmentation procedure. Int J Periodontics Restorative Dent 2001;21:561-7.

13. Schlee M, Steigmann M, Bratu E, Garg AK. Piezosurgery: basics and possibilities. Implant Dent 2006;15:334-40.

14. Toscano NJ, Holtzclaw D, Rosen PS. The effect of piezoelectric use on open sinus lift perforation: a retrospective evaluation of 56 consecutively treated cases from private practices. J Periodontol 2010;81:167-71.

15. van den Bergh JP, ten Bruggenkate CM, Disch FJ, Tuinzing DB. Anatomical aspects of sinus floor elevations. Clin Oral Implants Res 2000;11:256-65.

16. Becker ST, Terheyden H, Steinriede A, Behrens E, Springer I, Wiltfang J. Prospective observation of 41 perforations of the Schneiderian membrane during sinus floor elevation. Clin Oral Implants Res 2008;19:1285-9.

17. Peleg M, Chaushu G, Mazor Z, Ardekian L, Bakoon M. Radiological findings of the post-sinus lift maxillary sinus: a computerized tomography follow-up. J Periodontol 1999;70:1564-73.

18. Cortes AR, Cortes DN, Arita ES. Effectiveness of piezoelectric surgery in preparing the lateral window for maxillary sinus augmentation in patients with sinus anatomical variations: a case series. Int J Oral Maxillofac Implants 2012;27:1211-15.

19. Zitzmann NU, Schärer P. Sinus elevation procedures in the resorbed posterior maxilla. Comparison of the crestal and lateral approaches. Oral Surg Oral Med Oral Pathol Oral Radiol Endod. 1998;85(1):8-17.

20. Cho SC, Wallace SS, Froum SJ, Tarnow DP. Influence of anatomy on Schneiderian membrane perforations during sinus elevation surgery: Three-dimensional analysis. Pract Proced Aesthet Dent 2001;13:160-3.

21. Hallman M, Nordin T. Sinus floor augmentation with bovine hydroxyapatite mixed with fibrin glue and later placement of nonsubmerged implants: A retrospective study in 50 patients. Int J Oral Maxillofac Implants 2004;19:222-7.

22. Papa F, Cortese A, Maltarello MC, Sagliocco R, Felice P, Claudio PP. Outcome of 50 consecutive sinus lift operations. Br J Oral Maxillofac Surg 2005;43:309-13.

23. Hernandez-Alfaro F, Torradeflot MM, Marti C. Prevalence and management of Schneiderian membrane perforations during sinus-lift procedures. Clin Oral Implants Res 2008;19:91-8.

24. Aimetti M, Romagnoli R, Ricci G, Massei G. Maxillary sinus elevation: the effect of macrolacerations and microlacerations of the sinus membrane as determined by endoscopy. Int J Periodontics Restorative Dent 2001;21:581-9.

25. Katranji A, Fotek P, Wang HL. Sinus augmentation complications: etiology and treatment. Implant Dent 2008;17:339-49.

26. Hernandez-Alfaro F, Torradeflot MM, Marti C. Prevalence and management of Schneiderian membrane perforations during sinus-lift procedures. Clin Oral Implants Res 2008;19:91-8.

27. Vlassis JM, Fugazzotto PA. A classification system for sinus membrane perforations during augmentation procedures with options for repair. J Periodontol 1999;70:692-9.

28. Betts NJ, Miloro M. Modification of the sinus lift procedure for septa in the maxillary antrum. J Oral Maxillofac Surg 1994;52:332-3.

29. Beaumont C, Zafiropoulos GG, Rohmann K, et al. Prevalence of maxillary sinus disease and abnormalities in patients scheduled for sinus lift procedures. J Periodontol 2005;76:461-7.

30. Oikarinen K, Raustia AM, Hartikainen M. General and local contraindications for endosseal implants—An epidemiological panoramic radiographic study in 65-year-old subjects. Commun Dent Oral Epidemiol 1995;23:114-8.

31. Mardinger O, Manor I, Mijiritsky E, et al. Maxillary sinus augmentation in the presence of antral pseudocyst: a clinical approach. Oral Surg Oral Med Oral Pathol Oral Radiol Endod 2007;103:180-4.

32. Kara IM, Küçük D, Polat S. Experience of maxillary sinus floor augmentation in the presence of antral pseudocysts. J Oral Maxillofac Surg 2010;68:1646-50.

33. Celebi N, Gonen ZB, Kilic E, et al. Maxillary sinus floor augmentation in patients with maxillary sinus pseudocyst: case report. Oral Surg Oral Med Oral Pathol Oral Radiol Endod 2011;112:e97-102.

34. Tang ZH, Wu MJ, Xu WH. Implants placed simultaneously with maxillary sinus floor augmentations in the presence of antral pseudocysts: a case report. Int J Oral Maxillofac Surg 2011;40:998-1001.

35. Garg AK, Mugnolo GM, Sasken H. Maxillary antral mucocele and its relevance for maxillary sinus augmentation grafting: a case report. Int J Oral Maxillofac Implants 2000;15:287-90.

36. Zijderveld SA, van den Bergh JP, Schulten EA, ten Bruggenkate CM. Anatomical and surgical findings and complications in 100 consecutive maxillary sinus floor elevation procedures. J Oral Maxillofac Surg 2008 Jul; 66:1426-1438.

37. van den Bergh JP, ten Bruggenkate CM, Disch FJ, Tuinzing DB. Anatomical aspects of sinus floor elevations. Clin Oral Implants Res 2000; 11:256-265.

38. Cortes AR, Pinheiro LR, Cavalcanti MG, Arita ES, Tamimi F. Sinus Floor Bone Failures in Maxillary Sinus Floor Augmentation: A Case-Control Study. Clin Implant Dent Relat Res 2015;17:335-42.